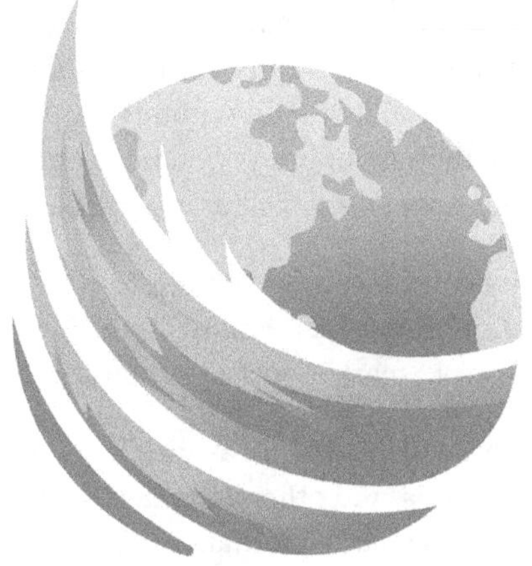

WAVE 4 HEALTHY LIVING

PRINCIPLES OF EXERCISE, NUTRITION, A HEALTHY MIND, AND A HEALTHY SPIRIT

By

Tom Wright

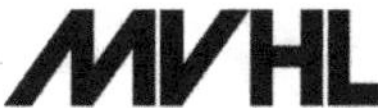

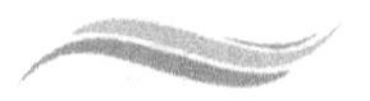

WAVE 4 HEALTHY LIVING

Principles of Exercise, Nutrition, a Healthy Mind, and a Healthy Spirit

For permission requests, write to the publisher, addressed
"Attention: Permissions Coordinator"
carol@markvictorhansenlibrary.com

Quantity sales special discounts are available on quantity purchases by corporations, associations, and others. For details, contact the publisher at carol@markvictorhansenlibrary.com

Orders by U.S. trade bookstores and wholesalers.
Email: carol@markvictorhansenlibrary.com

Cover Design - DBree, StoneBear Design
Book Layout - DBree, StoneBear Design

Manufactured and printed in the United States of America
distributed globally by markvictorhansenlibrary.com

MVHL

New York | Los Angeles | London | Sydney

ISBN: 979-8-88581-100-2 Hardback
ISBN: 979-8-88581-101-9 Paperback
ISBN: 979-8-88581-102-6 eBook
Library of Congress Control Number: 2023910115

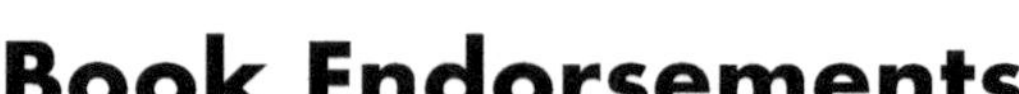

Book Endorsements

"I love the way Tom has integrated the body, mind, and spirit in this book. His message has broad appeal and will help those who read it to create more health, happiness and peace. The thoughts in this book are very similar to my own; which allow me to enjoy the wisdom of truth, beauty and love, in a youthful and active body. I would encourage all those who want to live a healthier and happier life to read Tom's book."

Grand Master Jhoon Rhee

- Speaker to United Nations (2007)
- Trainer of Muhammad Ali and Bruce Lee
- Father of Tae Kwon Do in America

***

"Our nation's health care crisis and the personal health tragedies and financial woes that result will only get worse until we as a nation start truly living healthfully. We can control our health destiny and win the war against heart disease and cancer but only by nutritional excellence, not more medications. I hope Tom Wright's new book is a huge success as it can curtail human suffering and save lives. "

Joel Fuhrman, MD

- 7X *NY Times* Best Selling Author
- Family physician
- Author of six books including, *Eat to Live*
- US World Figure Skating Team member

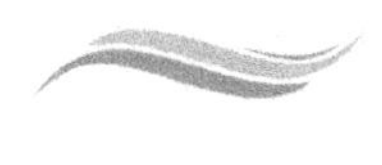

"Life for most of us as children and youth is centered on reacting to the instructions (verbal and observed) we receive from the authority figures in our lives, parents, teachers and others. If we are fortunate those influences are good, uplifting and enlightening. Frequently however, those important experiences of our "formative" years fall a bit short. Our maturity may be slowed or stopped because of lack of real direction about life's most important purposes and achievements. As Tom says in his book, "a person of 18 may be more mature than a person of 70." WAVE 4 Healthy Living is a comprehensive guide to living. The concepts in this book will help anyone live a healthy, happy, robust, fulfilling and righteous life. All who read it will find it informative, revealing, interesting and appealing."

Dr. L Jay Silvester

- Six-Time World Record Holder (Discus)
- Olympic Silver (Munich 1972) and Olympic Bronze Medalist (Montreal 1976)
- Retired College Professor
- Olympic Coach (Sidney 2000)

***

"I have known Tom for many years, I greatly admire his health, strength and skill, not only his body, but in all aspects of his nature. I would highly recommend this book to anyone who is interested in living a healthier life, especially for those like me who are up in age, and want to enjoy a high quality of life until the day they die."

Bob Engemann

- Member of the hit group, The Lettermen
- 32 Consecutive Billboard Magazine chart albums
- 11 Gold Records, 5 Grammy nominations, Andy Award, Cleo Award

Dedication and Acknowledgement

I humbly dedicate this book to all the great people in the world who have a desire to live healthier, happier lives—body, mind, and spirit!

I wish to acknowledge my indebtedness to the many people who have made this book possible. First, I want to thank my parents for teaching me the importance of education and good moral character. Second, I want to thank Dr. Barbara Lockhart, for her inspiring life and education, and her willingness to help me with this book. Dr. Lockhart is the Matriarch of WAVE.

I'm so grateful to Mark Victor Hansen, for his amazing accomplishments in life, and for choosing to publish this book, and to Mark's Executive Editor, Carol McManus, thank you for your great expertise in editing the manuscript and making it better than I could ever do on my own. David Lau is the illustrator for the Question Everything comics in the book, I'm so thankful for his great talent, and that we are friends. Next, I would like to thank my brother Robert and his family; Stacy, Cole, Bronson and Isabella, for their healthy example. I sincerely appreciate the other people who have helped prepare this book for publication, specifically, Melody Bates, and Flora Donaldson. I also appreciate and thank all my many friends, professional educators, and business associates.

People who I would like to thank specifically are: Ekaterina Rybakova, Dr. Gordon George, Maree Simmons, Robert and Julynn Simmons, Ken Porter, Dr. L Jay Silvester, Jeanne Hunter, Heath Jenni, Dr. Steve Cademartori, Dan VanVoorhis, Klark Keleman, Ray Weber, Keith Conley, Marie Krause, Salofi Hanneman, Melanie Schneiter, Kent Vorkink, Sheryl Lemke, Paul Engemann, Rex Vaughan, Stacey Hales, Jim Simmons, Brad Hoy, Kymra Donaldson,

Rhona Lopez, and many others. I can list so many others, but may I just say I am very blessed to have so many who have done so much to help me in my life. Many of you will never know how you have inspired me to press forward in times of trouble, to pick myself up when I fall, and to keep the faith and not give up on my dreams and desires in life. THANK YOU! This book is written out of my love and appreciation for my family and friends, and a desire to bless others as I have been blessed.

Most importantly I sincerely thank God, our Heavenly Father, and His Son Jesus Christ, for Their perfect love, guidance and direction. Notwithstanding my weaknesses, if you see anything that is good, right, and true in this book, it is a reflection of Them.

I hope you enjoy this book! If you have any suggestions or personal comments about how to make this book better, please write to me at QETommy@icloud.com.

Tom Wright

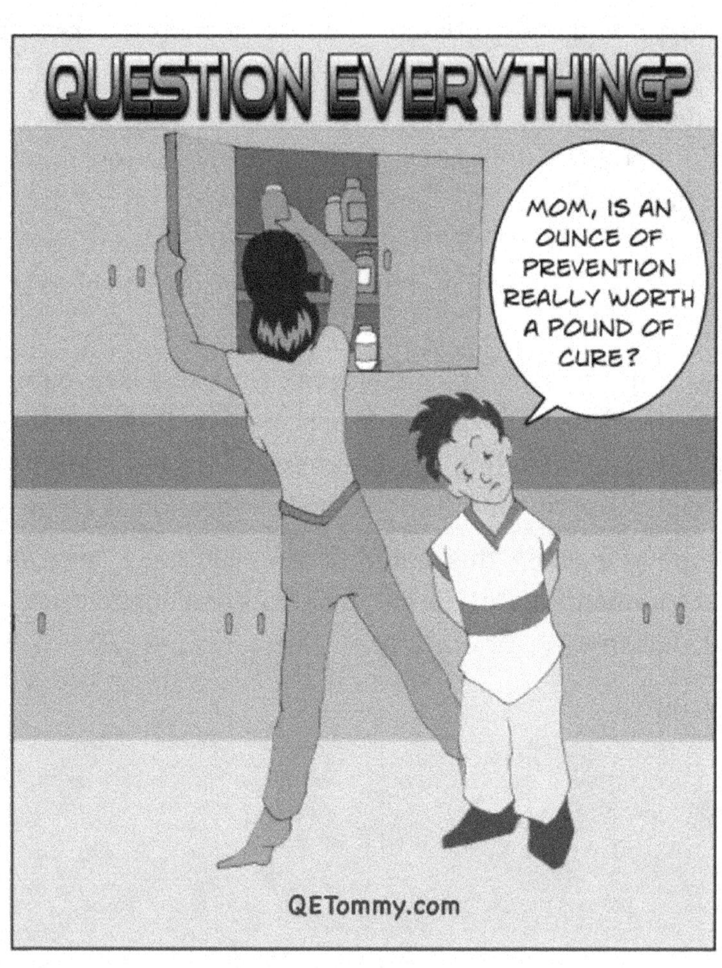
QUESTION EVERYTHING?
MOM, IS AN OUNCE OF PREVENTION REALLY WORTH A POUND OF CURE?
QETommy.com

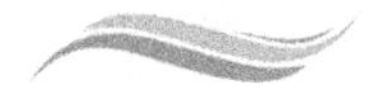

Table of Contents

Dedication & Acknowledgement VI

Introduction 1

7 PRINCIPLES OF EXERCISE 8

INTRODUCTION – 8

PRINCIPLE #1 – Evaluate Where You Are **11**
So You Know Where You Are Going

PRINCIPLE #2 – Catch the Wave! **14**
And You'll Be Sitting on Top of The World!

PRINCIPLE #3 – Do Something You Enjoy **22**
Train for a Purpose

PRINCIPLE #4 – Be Heart Healthy **29**
Both Aerobic and Anaerobic Will Do It

PRINCIPLE #5 – Whole Body Activities & Exercises Are Best **38**
Balance Your Body

PRINCIPLE #6 – Continually Change Your Workout **46**
Avoid plateaus, also mental and physical burnout

PRINCIPLE #7 – Use A BodyMindSpirit Approach to Fitness **53**
Anything less and you go in circles

7 PRINCIPLES OF NUTRITION 56

INTRODUCTION 57

PRINCIPLE #1 – Nutrition Is the Key to Health **60**
"The best medicine is food" –Hippocrates

PRINCIPLE #2 – Find Your Healthy Body Fat Level **69**
You are in control

PRINCIPLE #3 Free Radical/Ph Balance Theories **85**
Do we already know the cure for cancer?

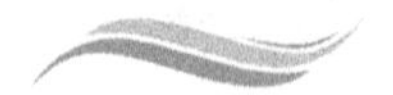

PRINCIPLE #4 Eat High Density Foods **104**

Is feeling satisfied, no obesity, and no disease really possible?

PRINCIPLE #5 – Words Of Wisdom **115**

There are many

PRINCIPLE #6 – Eat Foods Low on the Glycemic Index **128**

Keep your body fat low and your energy high

PRINCIPLE #7 – Use A Bodymindspirit Approach In Nutrition **141**

Anything less and you go in circles

7 **PRINCIPLES OF A HEALTHY MIND 143**

INTRODUCTION 144

PRINCIPLE #1 – Think And Grow Rich **145**

You are what you think about

PRINCIPLE #2 – Rely Upon God **158**

You cannot do it alone

PRINCIPLE #3 – Dream **161**

Make your dreams reality every day

PRINCIPLE #4 – Organize Your Life **166**

Create a proactive mind

PRINCIPLE #5 – Become Financially Secure **185**

Set yourself free

PRINCIPLE #6 –Work & Rest & Play **207**

Find the balance

PRINCIPLE #7 – Use A BodyMindSpirit Approach to Your Mind **217**

Anything less and you go in circles

7 **PRINCIPLES OF A HEALTHY SPIRIT 219**

INTRODUCTION 220

PRINCIPLE #1 – Look to God **225**

He can make a whole lot more out of your life than you can

PRINCIPLE #2 – Realize Your Potential **237**
The worth of souls is great!

PRINCIPLE #3 – Love **244**
The two great commandments

PRINCIPLE #4 – Keep Yourself Clean **250**
Have a pure heart and clean hands

PRINCIPLE #5 – Focus On Your Family **258**
They will be your greatest source of joy

PRINCIPLE #6 – Serve Others **264**
You will be in the service of God

PRINCIPLE #7 – Use A Bodymindspirit Approach To Your Spirit **268**
Anything less and you go in circles

APPENDIX 270

Suggested Reading Material **270**

Wave 4 Fitness Evaluation **275**

Wave 6-Week Fitness Challenge **280**

Wave 4 Nutrition Analysis **296**

About the Author **309**

References **312**

QUESTION EVERYTHING?

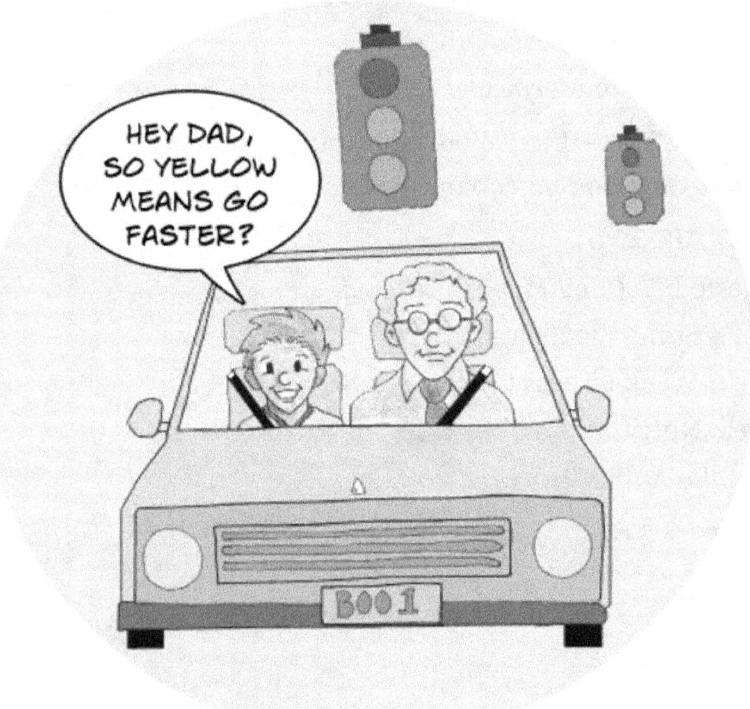

QETommy.com

Introduction

"To put the world in order, we must first put the nation in order; to put the nation in order, we must first put the family in order; to put the family in order we must first cultivate our personal life; we must first set our hearts right."

— Confucius

Currently America is in the middle of a "health care crisis." It is amazing to listen to all the discussion, with little or no mention of prevention. Yes, we need to lower health care costs, make sure our seniors are taken care of, cut out the waste, and make insurance available to the 30 million Americans who in 2021 were uninsured[1]... but other than running a more efficient health care system, the only other way to solve our health care crisis is to *help people to be healthier*. Amidst all the discussion, have we forgotten the most important ingredient?

The purpose of this book is to help you achieve more in your life and become a healthier, happier person! As you read this book and apply these basic principles to your life, you will find more health, happiness, and peace.

"For him who embarks on the path of seeking knowledge, Allah will ease for him the way to paradise."

—Abu Hurayrah

Isn't this what all of us really want the most in life?

Few will argue with the virtues of these principles, yet many have strayed far away from them. As you come to better understand them (we're all learning) and discover how to most aptly apply them to your

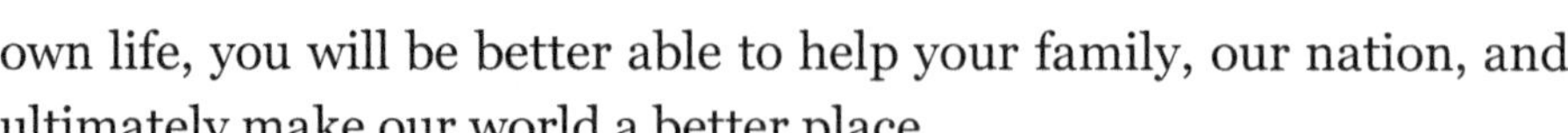

own life, you will be better able to help your family, our nation, and ultimately make our world a better place.

A principle might be best described as the following:

"A principle is an enduring truth, a law, a rule you can adopt to help you in making decisions. Generally, principles are not spelled out in detail. That leaves you free to adapt and find your way with an enduring truth, a principle, as an anchor.[2]"

—Boyd K. Packer

The focus will be the underlying principles that, if followed, normally result in great health.

The objective here is to teach correct principles, to hopefully help you live a better life; to educate rather than dictate. Greatly honored in this book is your freedom of thought and expression, your amazing mind, your likes and dislikes, the great talents you possess, everything that makes you unique and different from everyone else. While underlying principles are the main thrust of this book, some basic practices are included as well.

Your unlimited potential will be discussed at length; the hope is that as you truly understand your potential you will be able to push through the pitfalls, and distractions, and be all that you can be.

"What a piece of work is man! How noble in reason! How infinite in faculty! In form and moving, how express and admirable! In action, how like an angel! In apprehension, how like a god!"

—William Shakespeare

Prepare yourself as you read by keeping an open mind; open to inspiration, wisdom, understanding, and discernment of truth.

Then apply these principles to see if they work for you. As you follow true principles you will reap decided benefits, one of which is a greater sense of freedom.

Incorporated in this work is the wisdom of the ages through

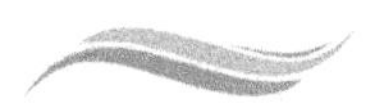

scientific research, great minds of past and present, logic, and scripture. This book is founded on a search for truth. These principles are the basics of life. They are time-tested truths that work. They are built upon solid foundations and are not the quick fixes or fads of the moment that we may find elsewhere.

The discussion will focus on principles that are geared more toward health than vanity. Many programs offer quick fixes that have little or no long-term success, while others produce amazing results but are simply not healthy. These principles, if adopted, will help you live a healthy and happy life. You might not look like a body builder, but you will be *healthy and attractive*. This is the focus.

Some principles are more important than others. Some have eternal significance, and others are only true for a moment in time. The principle of work (effort) and reward is eternal. If we put in the work, sooner or later we will reap the rewards of our efforts. The need to supplement is an example of a principle that might only be true for a moment in time. A hundred years ago most of us could probably get everything we needed nutritionally from our food supply. Most of our food was planted in healthy soils, it was not processed, and our air was clean and free of pollutants. Today it is very difficult to get everything we need strictly from our food supplies. Hopefully, in the future things will change as we work to clean up pollutants and create healthier soils. In the meantime, we might need to enhance our food supply with supplementation.

What makes this book different from others about healthy living and self-improvement? First, many authors have focused mostly on just one or two aspects of our natures; many have done a great job with the body but have virtually ignored the mind and spirit. Others have done a great job with the mind and spirit but have ignored the body.

Understanding the reality of BodyMindSpirit wellness will help us enjoy a harmonious integration of our whole selves. If an ailment

afflicts our body or mind, it will affect all of us, not just individual parts. This book addresses all aspects of our nature.

This book also simplifies basic concepts and breaks them down into understandable principles, and a whole company is built around this book and these principles. In January of 2000 WAVE was founded. **WAVE** represents ***W**orldwide **A**chievement, **V**itality & **E**xcellence*. This gives you a company family to go to for help, or just a place to meet people with common interests.

WAVE's main company website is wave4life.com, from it you will be directed to all our other websites, services and products. In the past we had a national TV show about healthy living that ran into 50 million American households on mainstream TV entitled ***GAGA 4 Healthy Living*** that we hope rebrand as ***WAVE 4 Healthy Living*** and get it back on the air soon.

We are working on social, business, and networking sites that give you a place to meet others that are interested in healthy living. Also, a site for healthy-minded singles, a fitness site to help you take optimal care of your physical body and train for specific activities or objectives, a nutrition site for those interested in improving their nutrition, having more energy, losing weight, and becoming healthier, a coaching site for those who are looking for personal coaches who help in a variety of areas, such as certified financial planners, marriage and family therapists, personal development coaches, personal trainers, and registered dieticians, a talent website devoted to developing talent in a variety of disciplines, including models, actors, and entertainers. Entertainers include musicians, singers, dancers, comedians, bands, and artists. We also plan to have athletic apparel and a sport accessories line, and a pure and natural line of personal care products.

WAVE's mission is to bring you the very best products and services available in health and wellness.

This book is separated into four main sections: Exercise, Nutrition,

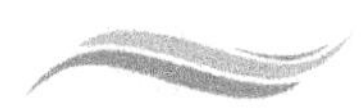

Mind, and Spirit. In each of the four main sections 7 basic principles of healthy living are presented. In WAVE we plan to have people enter coaching sessions to focus on improvement and achievement in each of the 4 main areas, which is the reason the book is organized this way.

The body (fitness & nutrition) is considered first because of our nation's health care crisis, also because this is often people's greatest area of interest. People are always concerned about their health; they want to look good and feel better. This book will help you in your quest to become a healthier, happier person.

Also included are some Question Everything Comics. Enjoy them!

I love you and sincerely appreciate your time and attention!

Cheers! ☺
Tom Wright

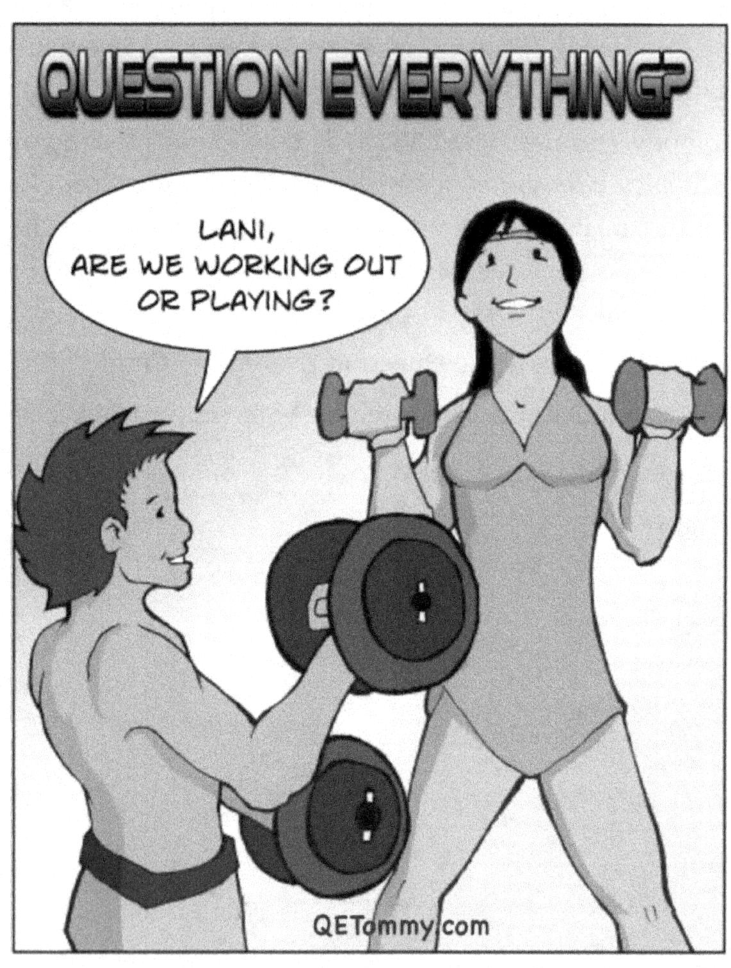
QUESTION EVERYTHING?
LANI,
ARE WE WORKING OUT
OR PLAYING?
QETommy.com

7 PRINCIPLES OF EXERCISE

"The Master in the art of living makes little distinction between his work and his play, his labor and his leisure, his mind and his body, his education and his recreation, his love and his religion. He hardly knows which is which. He simply pursues his vision of excellence in whatever he does, leaving others to decide if he is working or playing. To him he is always doing both."

—Zen Buddhist Proverb

INTRODUCTION

The purpose of the 7 Principles of Exercise is to help you live a healthy, happy, and productive life.

Exercise is a wonderful thing. It is something that makes us feel good, glad to be alive. From the day we are born until the day we die movement is an important part of life. If we are physically active throughout our lives we can live a rich full life, open and receptive to all of life's challenges and joys, develop our great talents, and avoid most of the problems associated with poor health or injury.

Exercise includes anything where we move our body. It can be something as simple as standing up from a chair, or walking out to the mailbox, to something as challenging as playing professional baseball or running a marathon.

As in the other sections, basic principles are identified which, if incorporated, will open your life up and help you to live a more enjoyable and productive life. These principles are not new, but they are not understood or practiced by most. They make sense and are easy to understand and apply to your life; but to truly appreciate them and use them to open your life up it will require sincere effort on your part. Once you internalize these principles, they are yours, and nobody will ever be able to take them away from you. They will bless you, and those you teach them to, for generations to come.

"There are some things which cannot be learned quickly, and time, which is all we have, must be paid heavily for their acquiring. They are the very simplest things, and because it takes a man's life to know the little new that each man gets from life is very costly and the only heritage he has to leave."

—Ernest Hemingway

There is not a lot of opposition to exercise; most people agree that anything we do to move our bodies, unless done in excess, is good for us. The challenge comes from complacency, resistance to exercise, or just figuring out how best to train. Some think they do not have the time, or just lack the desire to exercise or train hard for a sport.

These principles, if followed, will make exercise fun again. They will help you to see the importance of exercise to a healthy and productive life and arm you with the necessary knowledge and power to break down the walls of resistance, or just help you to know how to train smarter.

Exercise relieves stress, helps our bodies to function properly, prevents illness and disease, helps keep the body fat off, it releases the same chemicals in the brain as an anti-depressant, it makes muscles toned and hard, it prevents injuries, it helps us think clearly, it has no harmful side effects, it creates better athletes, it helps keep the zest and vigor of youth, it empowers our mind and spirit, it gives us

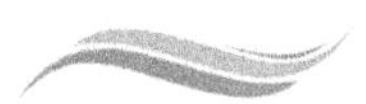

confidence and strength, it helps us develop our talents, it gives us freedom and a sense of accomplishment, it empowers us and helps us to be independent and successful, it can help build friendships and unity, it helps make us attractive and appealing...exercise is a wonderful thing!

May this section help you to see the blessing it is to have a physical body. May it also help you to fine-tune your exercise and be all that you can be. May it be a guiding light and help show you the way.

Are you ready? Let's get started!

BEFORE WE START – please understand that before starting any exercise program you should have a physical examination by a licensed physician. If you have any physical limitations, injuries, or ailments, it is your responsibility to keep yourself free from serious injury or death.
Neither tom wright, wave international, wave fitness, nor any of wave's divisions or affiliate companies, officers, trainers, coaches, or independent contractors will be held responsible for any injuries or deaths. These principles are founded on a search for truth, but it is up to you to use good judgment and wisdom as you apply them to your own personal situation.

QUESTION EVERYTHING?
DAVID, SHOULD WE FIGURE OUT WHERE WE ARE AT, SO WE KNOW WHERE WE ARE GOING?
QETommy.com

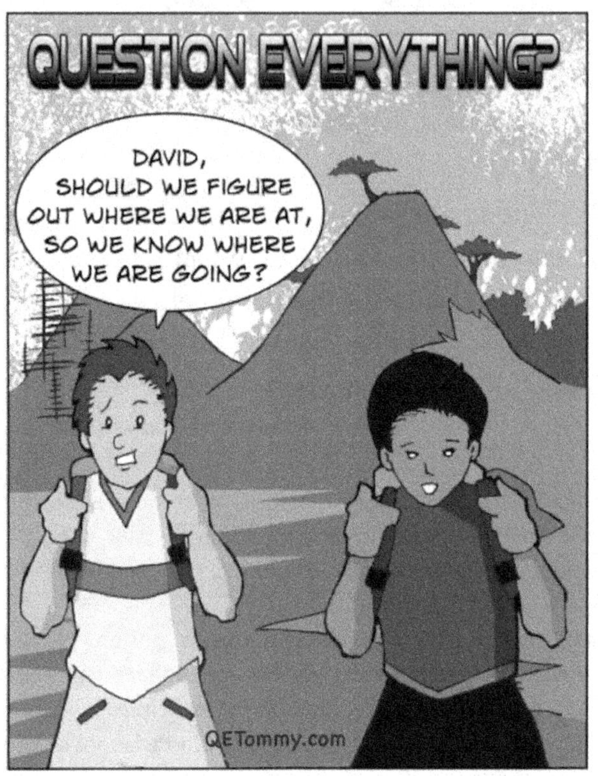

PRINCIPLE #1
Evaluate Where You Are At

So, you know where you are going

It is very important for you to complete the Fitness Evaluation before you start exercising. (See the Appendix) It is tough to know where you are going and how much progress you are making if you have no idea where you are currently at with your physical health.

"When performance is measured it improves."

—Thomas S. Monson

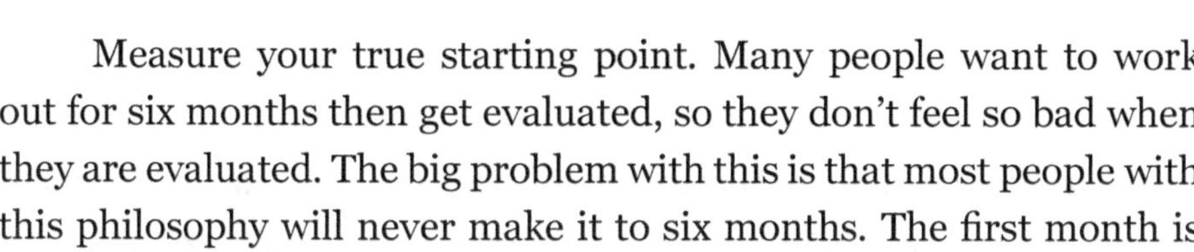

Measure your true starting point. Many people want to work out for six months then get evaluated, so they don't feel so bad when they are evaluated. The big problem with this is that most people with this philosophy will never make it to six months. The first month is critical to the success of anyone starting an exercise program. If you get evaluated and get a true starting point, you will:

1. **Recognize Your Strengths and Weaknesses** – Evaluate your body fat, cardiovascular capacity and conditioning (approximate VO2 Max), upper and lower body strength, resting heart rate, blood pressure, stomach strength, flexibility, and girth measurements. If possible, you are also encouraged to get your blood work done (cholesterol, HDL, LDL, triglyceride levels). Then compare these values to some of the charts that are gathered in the Appendix on averages for age groups and gender.[3] This will give you a good idea of where you are in comparison to the average American.

NOTE: Again, it is strongly recommended that you get a physical examination by a licensed physician before starting any exercise program. This fitness evaluation in no way replaces a physical examination by a doctor.

2. **Realize You Need Improvement in Your Health** – This evaluation is very motivating; it's been seen over and over again. You will get competitive with others and yourself. You may get disgusted or angry with yourself. You will take a serious look at yourself and where you are headed. Maybe you will remember back to when you were in good shape and how good you felt and how good you looked. Most importantly, you will be more motivated to improve.
3. **Recognize You Likely Need Help in Your Quest** – You have done it by yourself and look where you are. If you are in great shape, you are to be congratulated! But most aren't. If you are an average American, you are in trouble. If you come out average or below, maybe it is time to change your ways?

You can do better! If you need help visit us at **wave4life.com.**

4. **You Will Be Motivated by Your Improvement** – If you have a true starting point, when progress is made, which will be immediate, you will become more motivated. You will get excited! Most likely you will not be able to wait until your next workout. You will feel young again. You will feel more attractive. There is something about exercise, something that is hard to explain, something that makes us feel good, excited to be alive.

When you look in the mirror and see progress, you will get excited. When you measure your body fat and it is decreasing, see your heart healthy measurements improving, and you realize that you will live a longer, healthier, happier life, you will be excited. When you get stronger and your body gets toned in all those hard-to-get areas, you will get excited. And when you get excited you will change your lifestyle. Measure your progress and start with a true starting point, so you can look back in six months or a year from now and see how much progress you have made.

NOTE: See the Fitness Evaluation at the end of this book for the necessary forms, charts, and methods to complete the evaluation.

QUESTION EVERYTHING?
HEY LANI, WHAT CAUSES THE WAVES?
QETommy.com

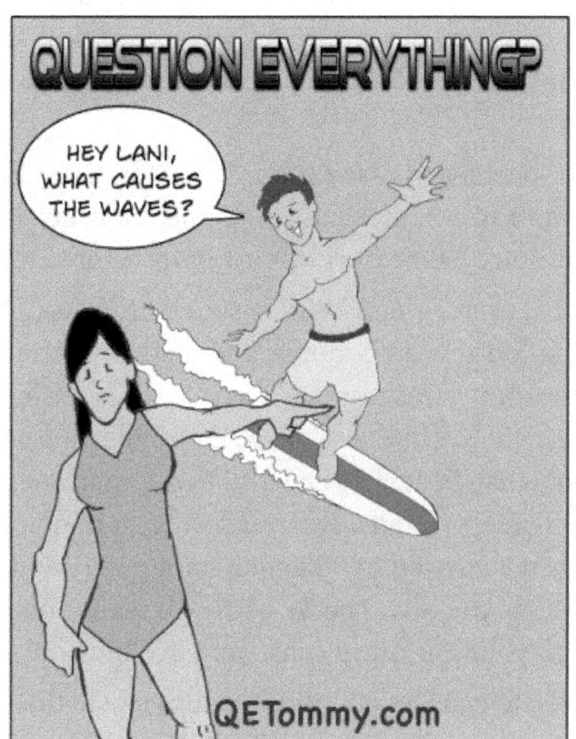

PRINCIPLE #2
Catch The WAVE!

...and you'll be sitting on top of the world
—Beach Boys

The ***WAVE*** is a new and improved way to exercise. It involves getting your heart rate up and then down, and then back up and then down...in a ***wave-type*** pattern. A couple decades ago research taught us that the best form of exercise was steady state or continuous exercise.[4] This research kicked off the aerobics craze of the 70's, 80's and beyond.

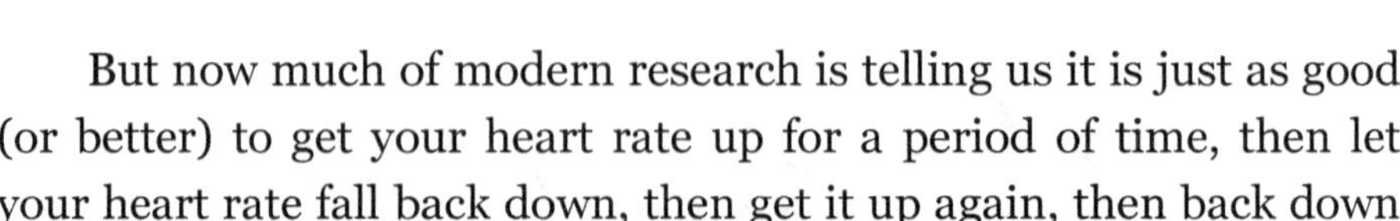

But now much of modern research is telling us it is just as good (or better) to get your heart rate up for a period of time, then let your heart rate fall back down, then get it up again, then back down (***WAVE***).

Instead of pushing yourself for 30 to 45 minutes, break up your exercise time into 10-minute chunks.[5] Using the heart monitor, bring your pulse rate down below 100 beats a minute before exercising again.

This form of exercise makes more sense. Many people come from a stressful situation at work or home, and then do continuous exercise and create constant stress on their bodies. Exercise helps relieve stress, but not if you push yourself hard the whole time without letting your body rest. It can be this way even at night; many never really give themselves a chance to wind down or allow their minds and bodies to relax. Not only do we need to take time out to relax and rest; we also need to learn *how* to relax. The ***WAVE*** will teach you how to relax, get in tune with your mind and spirit, and live life fully.

Doctors relate many of our physical ailments in the United States to stress.[6] Stress also creates an acidic pH in our bodies, which is a ripe environment for cancer and other diseases (see the Nutrition Principles).[7] Thus, it makes perfect sense why we have so many more health problems if we are stressed out so often. If we exercise using the WAVE, we will learn how to relax and get our heart rates down.

"Recent studies have concluded that stress is the cause of 80% of all diseases. Stress triggers the release of cortisol and adrenalin, which are both degenerative hormones. These contain the waste products called free radicals, which are now believed to be the leading cause of aging, cancer, and disease. Therefore, if we can handle greater amounts of stress without your body responding to it as an emergency, then we'll have made a huge dent in the war against aging and disease."

—John Douillard

The WAVE puts you more in touch with your whole self, body, mind, and spirit. It is suggested that you use a heart monitor when you exercise. Monitors start at about $35 and go up from there for the fancier ones. Some prefer the ones without a chest strap, so you can wear them as a watch and touch the face at any time for your heart rate. Others prefer the ones with the chest strap because you don't need to touch them to get the reading, which might make it easier to get your reading while you are exercising. Some watches now have heart monitors. You can pick up a heart monitor from WAVE through, wave4life.com (it is drop-shipped to your doorstep), or you can pick one up at most sporting goods stores.

One of the benefits of using a heart rate monitor is you will be less likely to stress your body out. When you go to the gym or exercise outdoors always check your heart rate before you exercise. If you don't have a heart monitor, take your pulse on your carotid artery (neck) or on your radial artery (wrist). If your pulse is elevated, back off your workouts, do something light or nothing at all. If you push yourself when your resting heart rate is elevated most likely you will add too much stress to your life, which will decrease your desire to exercise. Even though your body feels okay, it might be fighting off disease or just be tired.

A great idea might be to have a relaxation session instead of a workout on days when your resting heart rate is elevated. What a concept! Most times you won't get sick the next day or get so stressed out like you did before when you pushed yourself. Other times you might feel tired and sluggish, but your heart rate will be low. If you push your body hard you will likely feel fine the next day. You might feel sluggish because you slept too much, or your body's biorhythms might be off. Tracking your heart rate puts you more in touch with your body, mind, and spirit.[8]

In many of our youth sports kids get burnt out and never compete again after a young age. Why do so many put so much pressure on

kids that they end up hating what it is they are doing, or they end up quitting? Why do coaches make the workouts so long, hard, and boring? Why not mix in some other types of training or sports? Why do the sprinters and distance people many times do almost the same exact workout? Why do kids sometimes spend 3-5 hours training for a sport each day? People do not reach their physical peaks until their late 20's or 30's, some even do their best in their 40's...then why so much pressure on kids at such young ages?

How does this relate to you and the WAVE? Learn how to relax and pace yourself. Do not make your workout so intense you do not want to do it. Make it enjoyable. You might be saying to yourself, how can working out be enjoyable? When you truly understand the benefits of exercise, desire to develop your talents, and do exercise and activities you enjoy, it will be fun...even if there is some pain involved.

Tom's Testimony of the WAVE

"When I first started using the ***WAVE*** I was in college. I learned about it from my Professor, Dr. Barbara Lockhart, and she has written a whole book about it, Cardio Waves, read it! My resting heart rate was about 62, and within three months my resting heart rate was down to 52. I had a ten beat per minute improvement in three months! That means that every day my heart beats 14,000 times less than it did before. That is 100,000 less beats per week, and almost 5,000,000 less beats per year. If our heart has only so many beats in it, as some suggest, I will live approximately 14 years longer because I lowered my heart rate by ten beats per minute, if I keep my heart rate this low."

A good way to get your true resting heart rate is to measure it on your carotid artery in your neck, or on your wrist (thumb side) as soon as you get up in the morning. Because of medications and poor health, some people have resting heart rates over 100. The challenge for you is to see how much you can lower your pulse rate. There are some

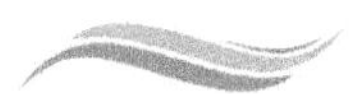

people in the world who, with concentrated effort, make their heart slow down to around 30 beats per minute.[9] As far as exercise and your heart rate goes; generally, the lower your heart rate the better shape you are in. Your heart is a muscle. The better conditioned or stronger your heart is, the less work it needs to do to supply your body with its needed oxygen and nutrients.

Another thing you will notice in your workout when using the WAVE is you will be stronger. When you lift, run, or do a physical activity, instead of walking around to keep your heart rate up, sit down, even lie down to get your heart rate as low as possible. When your heart rate bottoms out, then go ahead and do your next set or activity. Because you are more rested you will be stronger and have more energy, so you will be able to perform better in your workout or training session. You will have better workouts and teach your body how to relax at the same time! Better workouts will lead you to better performances.

You will also have a much better idea of how long to take between sets or activities, and how long your workouts should be. The Bulgarian weightlifters are arguably the best in the world. They say your body can only handle maximal output for about 45 minutes at a time.[10] So, they schedule 3-5 workouts a day, no more than 45 minutes at a time, with rest, food, and play in between. You will notice when using the WAVE that at the beginning of your workout your heart rate drops significantly faster than it does during the end of your workout, because your body is more fatigued at the end of a workout.

Many people like to take a certain time in between their sets, say a two or three-minute rest. A two-minute rest at the beginning of the workout might seem like a lot depending on what you are doing, but toward the end it might not seem like enough. If you feel like it is not enough rest, then it is likely not. If your body is tired, you need more rest. Listen to your body. If you do not give it the rest it needs, your performance will always be lacking. If your performance is lacking in

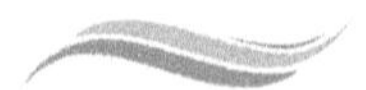

practice, it will be lacking in competition, because you play like you practice.

One of the most common problems in sports today is over training.[11] Sometimes athletes overdo, but often they do not rest enough between activities. More cross training can help to avoid mental and physical burnout. Cross training involves doing other sports or activities that complement your own sport or activity. This could be weight training for sprinters, or basketball for football players. Some athletes have spent three to five hours a day in college for four years practicing a sport but never improved...something is drastically wrong to spend this much time at something with little or no improvement. *If you are not improving, you are doing something wrong*. The heart rate monitor will put you more in touch with your mind and body, so this doesn't happen to you. If your heart rate is elevated and you are having a hard time getting it down, it is probably time to hit the showers or take a break, maybe do some stretches and go home.

Don't view this counsel as saying you should work out less than your competition. However, if the quality is high enough, the quantity might not be as important. Try to work harder and smarter and keep it fun. Instead of doing a two-hour workout at night as others do, maybe get up early and do a 45-minute workout before school, take a class where you can get another 45-minute workout in during the day, then maybe work out with the team for only one hour at night. If you go all-out in your workouts you will get a half hour more of workout time in per day than most everyone else, and most likely your workouts will be of higher quality, because you will be more rested, and thus more eager to work hard. This will inevitably translate into better performances than your competition.

"Your first attempt at a new skill is most important, because you're forging a new pathway...Every time you let yourself practice movements incorrectly, you're getting better at doing it incorrectly. It follows that you want to repeat the correct movement pattern as much

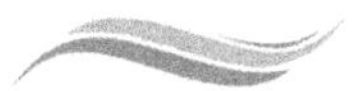

as possible to avoid, at all costs, reinforcing an incorrect pattern. A fundamental rule of learning, therefore, is never repeat the same error twice."

—Dan Millman

The importance of practicing when you are rested gives you a better assurance that you will be doing things correctly. Watch the best and copy them. They have proven their superiority. You do not need to reinvent the wheel, learn from them. For those of you who are not competitive athletes, these truths can be just as readily applied to your workouts or anything else you do in life.

If your goal is just to get in shape and feel good, maybe you can apply the WAVE by walking up and down the stairs at work five times a day with maybe an hour break in between. Or, instead of spending an hour and a half in the weight room a day, split that up and spend 30 minutes in the morning and 30 minutes at night. You will be amazed at the quality and quantity of what you can do in just 20 to 30 minutes.

Obviously, distance runners need to train for longer distances and keep their heart rates up for a longer time than the sprinters do. But by monitoring their heart rates when training, distance runners will have a better idea of how hard to push themselves. When their run is finished, then they can use the monitor to help them to relax and get their heart rate as low as possible. They can also use it more on their strength training days to become stronger, so they can hit those hills harder and have a better kick at the end of the race.

Another thing to mention here is the BodyMindSpirit approach to health and training. Smoking, drugs, some medications, obesity, lack of exercise, contention, lack of sleep, stress, and poor nutrition can all elevate your heart rate. It makes sense to monitor your heart rate to be more in tune with your whole self. If you truly want to be healthy and happy, you will eliminate these negative things from

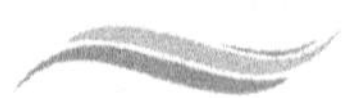

your life. This program focuses on your whole self, because a human being is not just a collection of individual parts. If you follow WAVE's complete program, you will improve and become better. Most of us are lacking in some critical areas in our lives, and all of us can make improvements in these areas.

QUESTION EVERYTHING?
MOM, HOW COME MOST KIDS STOP PLAYING WHEN THEY BECOME ADULTS?
QETommy.com

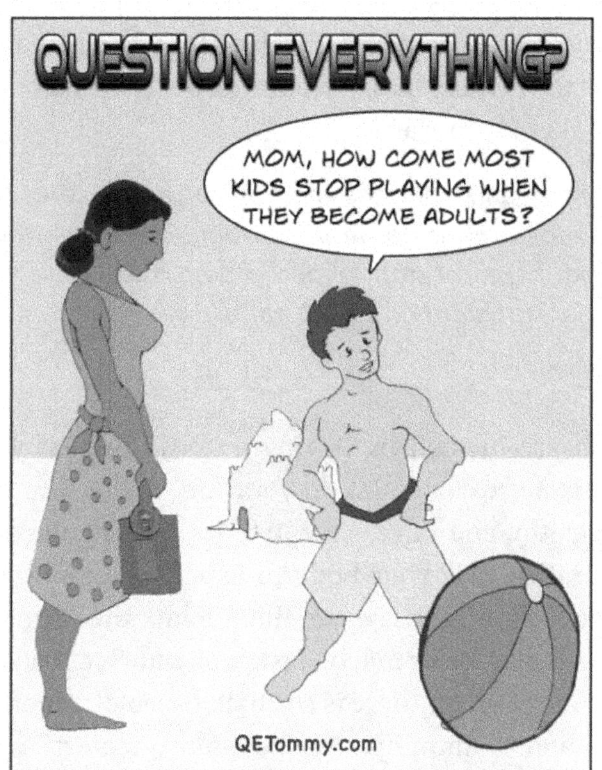

PRINCIPLE #3
Do Something You Enjoy
Train for a purpose

Get out and move your body! Do something you enjoy. Do something that motivates you to come back and do it again. Not everyone has to lift weights or play in a softball league or run a mile a day. Choose your activity and make it fun. You will be more productive, and happy, both at work and at home. WAVE is not a weightlifting program; we can set one up for you if you are interested. But the goal is to teach you how to live life optimally. WAVE will never try to force

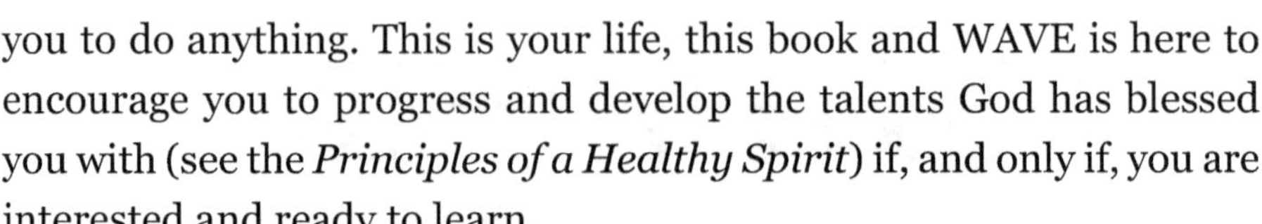

you to do anything. This is your life, this book and WAVE is here to encourage you to progress and develop the talents God has blessed you with (see the *Principles of a Healthy Spirit*) if, and only if, you are interested and ready to learn.

"Exercise programs enhance the job performance of adults and reduce the overall risk of many chronic diseases, particularly heart disease, hypertension, hyperlipidemia, obesity, mature-onset diabetes, osteoporosis, & certain types of cancer."

—Fitness For Life

We each are blessed by having a body. Even if your body is impaired, it is a great blessing to your life. You are responsible for keeping it healthy and alive, receptive to life and all its challenges and opportunities. Use your body to experience all that life has to offer. If basketball is your favorite thing to do, then play it. You may find a league to play in, or maybe just get a bunch of friends together periodically and play. Or there is softball, baseball, tennis, volleyball, racquetball, and swimming. Maybe your greatest asset is your physique, so you like to lift weights and compete in bodybuilding, or maybe you just like to lift to be toned and strong, or you may like to jog, and want to compete in a marathon? The important thing is that you do something, and it is suggested to do something daily. Riding bikes or roller blading is not just for kids. Why not join a league, or even a summer college league, if you think you still have it? Go see if those college kids can stay with you.

There is a great movie called *The Jericho Mile*. It is the story of a guy who was a mile runner and serving a life sentence in prison. They were going to let him compete in the Olympics and run the mile, then at the last minute they decided not to let him out. This about killed him. So, one day he went out with a stopwatch in his hand and ran the mile on the prison track. He broke the world record, with only the inmates looking on. After the amazing run, he threw the stopwatch

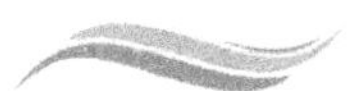

away. He did what he wanted to do and thought he could do. It did not seem to bother him much after that the world was not able to see him do it. What was important is he did it. Sometimes this will be the only satisfaction we will ever get in life. This earth life is not always fair. But, one day we will all be able to fulfill all our dreams, even if they do not come to pass during our lifetimes.[12]

If you can do something to fulfill your dreams now, do it. Why wait? Go after your own dreams, and do not live your life through your children or the television. Encourage your children to develop their own talents. Make everything available to them that you can. Expose them to a variety of activities when they are young, so when they get older, they can see for themselves where their greatest talents lie. Then let them choose. When they get to high school, maybe sooner depending on the activity, tell them that if they want to excel and take it to the next level, they need to focus in on what they want to do. The world is a competitive place. We might often feel like it is survival of the fittest, and if we measure everything in worldly terms it often is. So, encourage your children to focus, just not too soon so as to miss the wonders and enjoyment of childhood, or get burnt out and miss out.

Develop your talents. You are never too old. If someone tells you that you are, do not listen to those negative voices. Our nation needs more adult activities so we can develop our talents, be healthy, and not live our lives through our children. Example is the best teacher. In Japan businessmen play catch with a baseball on their lunch breaks. Why does sport or playing just have to be for kids? Take time to work out and play every day your whole life. One of WAVE's plans is to support and make people more aware of adult activities within their own communities, so they will participate themselves, have more balance and fun, and set the example for their children.

A great way to stay motivated and active is to train for a purpose. Remember specificity in your training.[13] Focus on baseball for baseball,

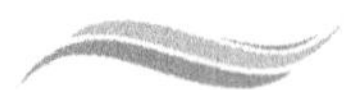

track for track, and weight training for bodybuilding. The best thing you can do to prepare yourself for a specific activity is to do that specific activity. You have to practice your sport or activity to get good at it.

Practice makes perfect. And most likely it is going to take some time to perfect what you are doing.

"An overnight success usually takes about ten years."

—Ben Hogan

So, work hard and be patient with yourself. Realize to be at the top of your sport, or to be the best you can be at anything, it will take time and much practice.

There was a famous pianist who said, "If I fail to practice for one day, I can tell the difference in my playing. If I fail to practice for two days, my family can tell the difference. If I fail to practice for three days, the world can tell the difference."

Having said this, there is most likely a point of diminishing returns in all sports or activities where you can only improve so much without increasing your strength, speed, size, flexibility, or doing some cross training. An example of this might be a sprinter who works out four hours a day at the track but has reached a point where their improvement is nominal, even with all this training. If others are training four hours a day on the track, it might be better to back off to 2-3 hours a day, or even less, and do other things like strength training in the weight room. That one hour a day in the weight room might allow a sprinter to improve their times more than if they spent that time out on the track. Why? There might be a lot of reasons. By increasing their size and strength in the weight room, especially if they can increase their power (strength/time), their sprint times should improve. Another reason for this improvement might be that the change of activity allows the person to avoid mental burnout so they can work harder during practice, or it might allow them more rest between activities. This is where a good coach comes in. Coaches

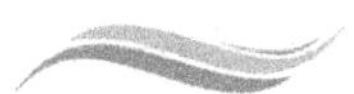

should be experts in dealing with their athletes and know when to change the activity to meet the needs of the athlete for both the short term and long term. This is what WAVE offers you; whether you are a competitive athlete or not, you can have your very own personal coach to guide you through your goals and objectives.

In the weight room people always ask if it is better to do slow controlled movements or fast quick movements. They ask if they should lift heavy weights or light. Should they do more repetitions or less? The answers depend on what you are trying to do. Get strong? Get toned? Get the fat off? Generally, the faster you move the weights, the more you will create power (strength/time) in your muscles.[14] Heavy weight with fewer reps will create strength, and if you increase the volume (more sets) in your workout, you will create more size in the muscle.[15] In Arnold Schwarzenegger's book, *Arnold's Bodybuilding for Men*, he talks a lot about getting a pump in the muscles, getting as much blood in them as possible through lots of sets, reps, and heavy weight.[16] If you want to get strong and hard but do not want to increase in size, do more weight, less volume (less sets), with more rest between the sets. Be careful not to move the weight too fast, because you can cause serious injury when you do jerky movements.[17] Slower, controlled movements with less weight, more reps, and less sets (volume) are better for people who are just starting out and are conditioning the tendons and ligaments.[18]

Decide what you want to accomplish and figure out the best way to get there. Have an objective in mind. Before training ask yourself what you want to accomplish. Do you want to become healthier, train for a specific sport, or look a certain way? Most people just want to lose fat and tone up their bodies. There is a continuum of physiques out there. At one end of the spectrum is the long-distance runner, and at the other end is the bodybuilder. Where on this continuum would you like to be? The bodybuilding end is distorted because many bodybuilders take drugs such as steroids. Even if you trained

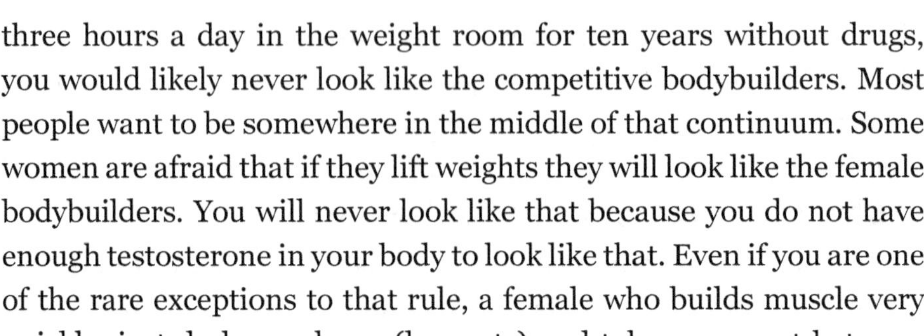

three hours a day in the weight room for ten years without drugs, you would likely never look like the competitive bodybuilders. Most people want to be somewhere in the middle of that continuum. Some women are afraid that if they lift weights they will look like the female bodybuilders. You will never look like that because you do not have enough testosterone in your body to look like that. Even if you are one of the rare exceptions to that rule, a female who builds muscle very quickly, just do less volume (less sets) and take more rest between sets and you will get toned and strong, but will not get bulky.

People generally want the same things in life when it comes to physical fitness. They want to look and feel good and want to be healthy. If your goal is to look more like the bodybuilders, then do more weight training, maybe 3-6 days a week. If your goal is to look more like a long-distance runner, than do more long distance-type work. It doesn't have to be running. Walking is better, unless you are an athlete training for something that requires running. Running is really tough on your body, especially if you are overweight. A recent article said that with every running step you put triple your body weight on your legs and joints.[19] So if you weigh 150 pounds that is 450 pounds of pressure with every step. If you do want to run because you are training for a marathon or a 5- or 10-K race, try to run more on soft surfaces like grass, than running on a hard surface like pavement. It is okay to run up hills that are hard surfaces, but do not train running down as you may risk injury to your knees. If you have to train on pavement, make sure you wear good shoes. If it's Nike you like, get the full air soles. These are typically over $100. The ones under $100 generally have just heel air soles. It is smart to buy them at an outlet store. You can often buy full air soles for under $50 at a Nike outlet store. Adidas, Reebok and New Balance also make great running shoes. Have someone who knows what they are doing help you pick out a good pair.

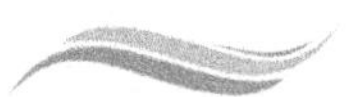

If your goal is something in the middle of the continuum, it is suggested that you do a combination of aerobic and anaerobic activity. Aerobic activity is activity in which you keep your heart rate up for an extended amount of time. Anaerobic activity is activity in which you exert yourself for short periods of time, generally for less than a minute. This leads us to the next principle.

QUESTION EVERYTHING?
MOM,
IS RUNNING OR JUMPING
BETTER?
QETommy.com

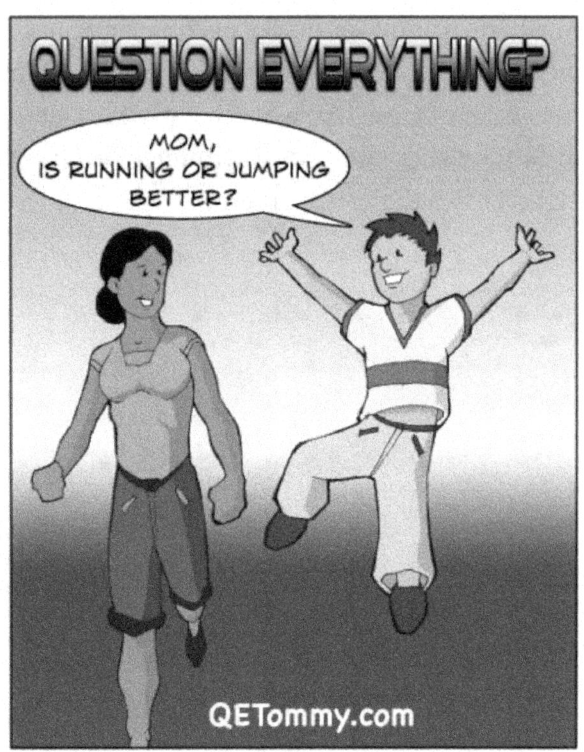

PRINCIPLE # 4
Be Heart Healthy

Both aerobic and anaerobic will do it

Aerobic conditioning, activity longer than 45 seconds, builds the *volume* of your heart; your heart actually gets bigger. Anaerobic conditioning, short bursts of activity less than 45 seconds, builds the *thickness* of your heart walls.[20] Your heart is a muscle. It needs to be exercised in order to remain healthy and strong. Activities like lifting weights, doing sprints, and running stairs, are generally anaerobic activities. You can turn them into aerobic activities by decreasing the

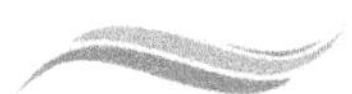

resistance (doing them very slow, light weight) and increasing the duration without much rest in between the set or activity. But anaerobic activities usually take so much effort and energy that you can only do them for a short time and then you need to rest. Aerobic activities can be done for long periods of time because you are not going all out. You pace yourself so you can go for extended periods of time. The time frame for anaerobic activity is usually about forty-five seconds or less.[21] This is the length of time that your body is capable of maximal output, after which you have to rest or you will be too tired to continue.

Much of the research in the past has centered on aerobic conditioning.[22] People thought the only way to have a good workout and build a strong heart was to keep your heart rate high for extended periods of time. With aerobic conditioning your heart volume increases, so you can pump more blood to your muscles with the same number of beats per minute. When you do anaerobic conditioning, your heart wall gets thicker so your heart can withstand stressful explosive movements and activities.

It's likely best to do both aerobic and anaerobic activity. Of course, it depends on what you are training for, but for overall health, a combination is your best bet. If you desire to do both, do an anaerobic strength-training program half of the time, and some type of aerobic conditioning the other half of the time. But make sure you do the activities you enjoy the most, because you will be much more likely to keep doing it. If you are into basketball, maybe you can play 2-3 times a week and lift weights 2-3 times a week. Or if you are into kickboxing aerobic conditioning classes, you can attend them 2-3 days a week and do stairs and hills 2-3 days a week. It's best if people do something physical every day.

If we do things every day, they get easier. Mix it up. Ride your bike, walk up and down the stairs a few times, play catch with your kids, race someone in a sprint, go for a swim. It is easier to do something every day because you get in the habit. It takes approximately twenty-one

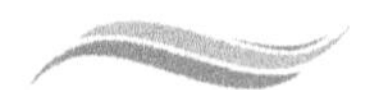

days to establish a habit.[23] If you do something every day, six days a week, you will be in the habit of exercise within three weeks (see the 6-Week Fitness Challenge - Appendix). You will start to feel better and look better in less than a month!

Our bodies crave exercise. If you want to feel vibrant and alive, exercise. Go move your body and do something you enjoy. Many people are so out of tune with their bodies that they have no idea what their bodies crave. People go on eating binges with no thought that their body might be lacking nutrition, so it is telling them to eat. They may feel sluggish, have no energy, be all stressed out and irritable, yet take no thought that their body might be begging for exercise. Get in touch with your body. Listen to it. Get in tune with the amazing instrument you've been given so you recognize what it is telling you.

Excuses for Not Exercising

TIME seems to be the biggest objection to exercise. Did you know you need less sleep, not more if you exercise regularly with prudence?[24] You will be less stressed out, create less free radicals, have a more alkaline pH in your body (see Principles of Nutrition), be healthier, be more productive and focused, look younger, and live longer?[25] Some people try this and say they need more sleep, not less. Well, give your body a chance to condition itself and pull some of the fat off. You will feel better, sleep better, have more energy, and eventually need less sleep, not more. Now, a competitive athlete who is spending 3-5 hours a day training obviously will need more sleep, not less, but most of us will never push our bodies this hard. Everybody, at least once in their lifetime, should train 2-3 hours a day for at least 6 months. This might be impossible for you right now, but accept this challenge sometime in your future, even if you are 90 years old when you do it. It is an amazing feeling to train this much. You feel so good, and you will never be comfortable again being out of shape. Our bodies are truly a blessing from above.

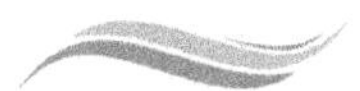

Parents often face the dilemma of not wanting to take time away from their families to exercise. Whoever said we need to? Take a child with you to the gym. Buy a walker for your child so you can take your children with you. What better way to set a good example for your children of a well-balanced, fit, and whole person. Example is the best teacher.

"Children have never been very good at listening to what their parents tell them – but they never fail to imitate them."

—James Baldwin

Chances are if you are healthy, they too will be when they grow up. If your children are too young to bring to the gym, take them to the park and have races with them. They love that active time together with you. Or just have them there with you at home when you exercise...time is no excuse.

CONVENIENCE is another big objection. If a gym is not within a convenient distance from your home or work, then get a few weights and create your own gym at home. See the Appendix for a suggested workout, or go to our website, wave4life.com, and view some home gym equipment options. You can start with very little expense, $100-$200. Obviously the more expensive equipment will take some money, but free weights are always better than machines, and they are relatively inexpensive.[26] Do some of the other suggested exercises and activities. You do not have to lift weights or go to aerobics classes to get a good workout and be fit. In fact, many times you can get a better workout at home or just as you go about your daily activities. Use the WAVE on a daily basis. Walk up and down stairs whenever you can. Forget about the elevator. Park your car far away from the store so you get more walking in, and don't get door dings in your car. Do a set of squats between doing the laundry or at the office. If you do not have any weights, just do the exercises without weights and do more repetitions. If you want toned buttocks, legs, or back, there is no better exercise than squats or dead lifts.[27] Convenience is no excuse.

LAZINESS seems to be a big reason why people do not exercise. Is it their fault people are lazy? Who really knows? We all have our free agency, but it is much harder for some than others. Maybe they were brought up that way with a bad parental example, so it seems like a waste of time or normal to not exercise. Maybe they have been on so many fad diets that their metabolisms are all messed up, or maybe they are so overweight that it is really miserable and seems useless to exercise, so they just give up. In come cases, people who have been abused physically or sexually, gain weight to subconsciously protect themselves from their perpetrators. We need to be very careful about judging other people. Our true understanding of others and their situation is so limited. The best thing we can do is to offer a helping hand. But, no more excuses. Go move your body!

To assure your heart healthiness use the WAVE in your training. If you have a heart rate monitor, use it every time you work out. Try to get your heart rate as low as possible between exercises or activities. See how low you can get your resting heart rate. You will most likely live a longer, healthier, happier life the lower you can get it. If something like coffee, cigarettes, drugs, lack of sleep, lack of exercise, or the inability to relax are elevating your pulse, then change your lifestyle. Get these things out of your life. Use the WAVE to put you more in touch with the amazing gifts you have been given.

How about for fat loss, which is better, aerobic or anaerobic? They both work.[28] Who knows which does the better job? One study says that one is better than the other, and another says the opposite. Again, it is likely best to do both. Think of your favorite activity or sport. Is it more aerobic or anaerobic in nature? If your physique is what you are working on, what kind of physique do you desire? Maybe you are a male and prefer to look more like the body builder than the long-distance runner. You might have the kind of body that is naturally thin, so to have some curves on your body you will need to lift weights. If you are training for sports like baseball and golf, anaerobic training

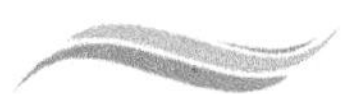

is generally much more effective. All the movements in baseball and golf are split second. They are highly explosive sports. This means a powerful athlete has a great advantage, especially in baseball. In golf it is not as big of an advantage to be big and strong and can even be a hindrance because "feel" is so important (if you get too big and strong you can lose feel). Both are highly skilled sports. In baseball you are hitting a round ball with a round bat, and the ball is traveling at 90 miles per hour. Ted Williams said hitting a baseball is the hardest thing to do in all of sport.[29] It not only takes skill and strength, but it takes strength over a short amount of time, which is the definition of power. In golf, flexibility and range of motion are more of a factor, and you are hitting a round ball with a semi-flat surface that is traveling about 100 miles per hour. Even though the ball is still, the margin of error is still very small, if you want it to go straight. Those of you who are golfers might be saying that hitting a golf ball is the hardest thing to do in all of sport! ☺

How does this relate to you? Does your favorite sport or activity involve split-second movements, long slow endurance movements, or a combination of both? Basketball is an example of something that is both. You need to be quick and powerful, but you also need to be able to run up and down the court for long periods of time. Remember specificity in your training. Also, remember your goals. Do you want some curves or just want to be thin? Most people want to be thin with tone to their muscles and a few curves here and there. First, get the fat off. You will never see your muscles or curves if you are covered with fat. Sometimes it's best to be clear and direct, so people understand. Remember, approximately 70% of fat loss is nutrition. Nutrition and exercise go hand in hand, like two oars in a rowboat. If pulling fat off is your main concern, focus on both healthy nutrition and exercise.

In order to burn fat doing aerobic exercise you will need to get your heart rate up for extended amounts of time. In aerobic training you can go for extended amounts of time because you are not going

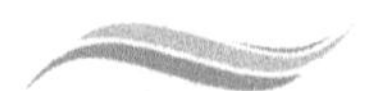

all out. It is generally recommended that you get your heart rate up to at least 60% of your max heart rate to get into your aerobic training zone.[30] This is not hard to do. Your max heart rate is 220 - age, so if you are 40 years of age, your max heart rate is 180 beats per minute.[31] Never get your heart rate above your max heart rate because you risk putting too much stress on your heart. You can easily check your heart rate with a heart monitor. It will calculate it for you. You can also take a quick measurement by checking your radial (wrist) or your carotid (neck) pulse. To get your heart rate for a minute, you can check it for six seconds and multiply your total by 10, just add a zero. So, if your heart rate is 12 for six seconds just add a zero and you get 120 for a minute. If you take it for 15 seconds, simply multiply it by four, for 30 seconds multiply by two.

So, if you are 40, your max heart rate is 180. Take 60% of that, 108, and you have your *aerobic training zone.* If you are 30 years old, your max heart rate is 220-30 (age) = 190, then times it by 60% and you get 114 for your aerobic training zone. If you are 60 years old, 220-60 (age) = 160 (max heart rate), times 60% gives you 96 for your aerobic training zone. You get the idea. Figure out where your aerobic training zone is at. Of course, you can train yourself aerobically below this "zone", but the idea is to get you to a point where you will really burn some calories and make a difference in your fitness and body fat levels. 60% of your max heart rate is easy to get to, but you have to do it for an extended period time to do much good. Most of the health resorts across the country help their clients lose weight very quickly because they put them on a good nutrition program and have them walk a couple hours a day. If people get their heart rates up into the aerobic training zone for 2 hours, which is easy to do, they are going to make a tremendous difference in their fitness level. Is it any wonder that people lose so much body fat in these programs?

Some people think they need to be panting to get in a good aerobic workout. The aerobic training zone is easy to achieve. It might

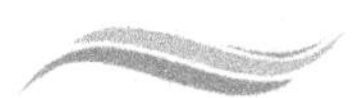

be a little uncomfortable at first if you go for long periods of time, but basically it is a comfortable exercise zone that just makes you breathe deeply.[32] You do not need to get your heart rate much above this deep breathing...duration is the key.

Now, some people get so caught up in this that they forget about the WAVE. It is easy to use the WAVE on your anaerobic days. Just rest and get your heart rate as low as possible in between your exercises or activities. On your aerobic days just do not rest as much between your sets or activities. Maybe do a run/walk, bike, or walk on hilly terrain, or do some stairs or wind spirits, and try not to let your heart rate get too low between sets.

Remember that anaerobic exercise builds muscle much better than aerobic exercise, and this muscle in turn burns fat off your body. The bigger the muscle, the easier it will be to get the fat off and keep it off. This is another reason many body builders take steroids or other drugs that make their muscles big. Big muscles make it easier to pull the fat off.[33] Now, the use of drugs is sure not being promoted here, on the contrary, but it does help to condition (tone) or build some muscle if you want to make it easier to maintain low body fat.

It would be good to say something here about *when* is the best time to exercise. It will depend on what you do during the day, but the general rule is when you are *best fed and most rested.*[34] You will most likely be best fed during lunch or dinner, and most rested in the morning. This might create a dilemma. If you are in a stressful work situation, the best time to exercise might be the mornings, but it is hard to get up early enough to fix a great breakfast, so you are best fed for your morning workout. If you work out in the morning and eat too close to a really hard workout, your blood sugar levels (your food supply in your blood) might still be low from the night without food, and if you exercise too close to food you might have an upset stomach because your food has not had time to digest. If you are in a good work situation, you can eat a big lunch so your blood sugar levels are

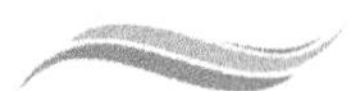

high (there is plenty of energy there for fuel). You will always be able to have a better workout if your blood sugar levels are high, especially if you are well rested. Nighttime is usually the hardest because you are tired from the day, but it is a great time to do your aerobic activity, because you do not need to use maximal output. Just keep going for an extended period of time with your heart rate just above 60% of your max heart rate (aerobic training zone) ...if your goal is fat loss.

It really all depends on your goals and your lifestyle. Just remember, you play like you practice, and if your practice is lacking, so will your performance. Another thing to consider is the presence or absence of training partners...generally you will always have more fun and train harder with someone else around. Factor this into your decision about when is the best time to train. This is one of the other beauties about having a personal trainer. They can generally be there with you whenever you need them. They can work around your schedule, not vice-versa.

QUESTION EVERYTHING?
LANI, DO YOU NOTICE THAT IF ONE OF US STOPS ROWING WE GO IN CIRCLES?
QETommy.com

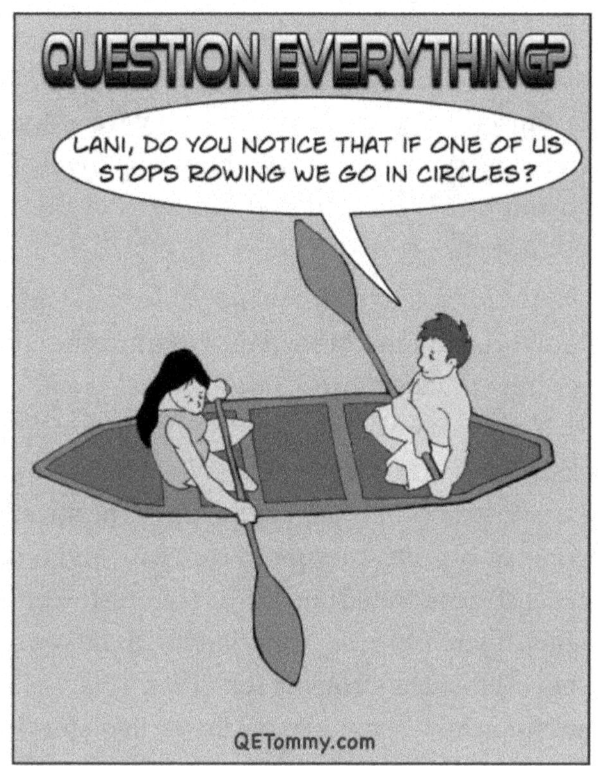

PRINCIPLE #5
Whole Body Exercises And Activities Are Best
Balance Your Body

If you want to do the best for your body in the least amount of time, you will focus on whole body exercises and activities. If time is your biggest objection to exercise, it is best to do things like dead lifts, squats, Pilates, and swimming. It would be good to do some of these anyway, and other activities or sports that exercise your whole body. You can do better in 10 minutes with these exercises and activities than 45 minutes doing less effective exercise.[35] Now, what about those

infomercials that advertise 3-5 minutes a day of whatever they are selling doing better for you than an hour a day in the weight room? It is mostly all nonsense. But when you do something like squats that hit virtually every muscle in your body with heavy weight, or swimming that does exercise every muscle in your body, you really can get more out of it in 10 minutes than doing 45 minutes of the less effective activity.

Many people do not like to swim, or do dead lifts or squats, because they hurt (good pain). More pain less time, the choice is yours. More pain less time makes more sense for most people, especially if they are busy. Your body will eventually thrive on the pain. It will make you feel alive, not in a sadistic way. Why? Because you know the pain will make you strong. It is a great feeling to be strong. When you bump into people or objects, they move, not you, and it does not hurt because your muscles are toned and hard. Your testosterone levels are also much higher if you exercise, especially with heavy weight.[36] Yes, that means you will have a stronger sex drive, which is a good thing if you are married. Unless you are on drugs like steroids, then just the opposite is true. Your body's natural production of testosterone shuts down, to accommodate the drug, the result being a significant decrease in your sex drive. We are meant to experience to the greatest degree all the wonderful feelings of life. Just make sure those feelings are directed through the proper channels and in the proper ways.

Focus on the biggest muscles in your body, which are your legs (quads and hamstrings), and glutes (your hind end). Then comes your back, stomach, chest, and shoulders, then finally your arms and calves. It is always amazing to watch people workout in the weight room. Some have really big chests and backs but have skinny legs. Often, they wear long pants to cover up their legs because they are embarrassed with them. Then there are people who have big strong arms, but everything else looks like they do not even exercise. If you are after overall health and symmetry, you will focus on the whole

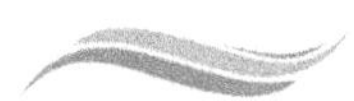

body, not just the parts. Just like it does not do much good to focus on the body and ignore the mind and spirit, it does not do much good to focus on specific parts of the body and forget about the whole.

If walking is your exercise, do not just walk on flat surfaces, walk up and down some hills or stairs. This will allow you to use the WAVE, as your heart rate will be higher walking up a hill, and lower walking down, and when you walk up hills you will exercise the back parts of your legs (hamstrings) and buttocks (glutes). This will firm up your butt! Who doesn't want that? ☺ If you walk only on flat surfaces, you will mostly work the front parts of your legs (quads), and it will be harder to use the WAVE in your exercise routine and achieve the results you desire. The same goes for running. Run up the hills so you work your hamstrings and glutes and walk down the hills. It is really hard on your knees to run down hills or stairs. What about your upper body? Maybe alternate with a strength-training program, or if you really do not like weight training, think of something you can do for your upper body. Maybe take some small hand weights with you as you walk, do some punching bag work (it is great for stress), do push-ups and pull-ups, play a sport that uses your upper body like golf, lift your kids up in the air every day...do something for your upper body.

One of the things that is so great about strength training (weights) is you can actually change the appearance of your body. If you have a skinny chest, you can make it bigger naturally. If you have narrow shoulders, you can get them looking toned and rounded. If you have a flat bottom (glutes) you can make it rounded and symmetrical. You can literally change your appearance. Not that our outward appearance is so important, but it is nice, and healthy, to be your best self physically and feel attractive. We have a responsibility to do all we can with what we have been given here on earth (see Principles of a Healthy Spirit), and this includes our physical bodies. Most people just do not know *how* to do it. This is the purpose of WAVE, to teach you how to be your best self, body, mind and spirit.

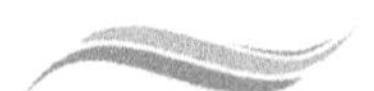

Most sports use your whole body. This is why athletic activities are so good for us and why it's a great thing for people to participate in sport. In the gym it's best to focus on whole body activities, things like squats, dead lifts, cleans, anything where the weight is placed on your upper body and you have to bend down into a squatting position to complete the movement. If you do not squat down all the way past parallel (parallel means that when you go down into the squatting position your upper leg is parallel with the floor—see wave4life.com for the online exercise videos), you will only be using your quads, and will cheat some of the biggest muscles in your body, your glutes and hamstrings. Many people like to do squats with a lot of weight, but don't go down to parallel. This will mainly only work the quads. It is better to back off the weight and go all the way down to parallel.[37]

SPECIAL NOTE: Be very careful when doing squats, deadlifts, cleans or other movements in the gym. you can seriously injure your knees and/ or back. make sure when performing these exercises you start with light weight, or none at all, and make sure you have correct form. see wave4life.com for correct form on squats, deadlifts, and other lifts. wave international, wave fitness, or any of its divisions or affiliates, officers, employees, trainers, or independent contractors will not be held responsible for any injuries or deaths. also have a spotter who knows what they are doing for any squat or bench press type movement, especially when the weight gets heavy.

Do not let the above warning scare you off from these exercises. Just realize it is your responsibility to keep yourself free of injury or death. If you do squats or any other movement with light weight, the risks are minimal. If you squat with just your body weight, it is the same movement as getting out of a chair, there is virtually no risk of injury, and we need to be able to do this movement till the day we die. If you strengthen your body, you will be less prone to injury, not more, because your body will be strong. Just work into things gradually and review the online videos for proper form, and you will be fine.

In many aerobic classes the instructors have the participants do many exercises but rarely have them bend down far enough to work the hamstrings and glutes ...these are two of the biggest muscle groups in our body, but across the board they are probably the most neglected. The best classes for you physically will focus on your largest muscles. Now, do not think it is a bad class just because they do not have you squatting down. There is a lot more to exercise classes than the optimal physical benefits. Did they motivate you to come back? Did you enjoy it? Did you get your heart rate up? If you attend an aerobics class where they neglect these muscle groups, just sell your instructor this book! ☺

What good is it to work out if you always get injured, do not really improve your health much, or never look any better? Any exercise is good, but some exercises are definitely better than others. We talked earlier about whole-body exercises being the best thing you can do. This is why sport is so good. Usually, you work your largest muscle groups in sport (your legs), and you get in competitive situations where you push a little harder and make it all more fun. At least it should be. Continual improvement and enjoyment are worthy goals. The other person is there just to have fun with...**T**ogether **E**veryone **A**chieves **M**ore (**TEAM**).

If you are weight training, focus on your core lifts (see Appendix). These are lifts that are typically whole-body lifts (like squats) where you can get the best results for your efforts (time). The other thing these lifts provide is good body balance. Core lifts work almost every muscle in your body.[38] If there is a weakness in your body these lifts will find it, sometimes to your detriment. So be careful you do not injure yourself. Start light and work up slowly. Your auxiliary lifts are the supplemental lifts that will add variety to your workout. These should change each month and be things you like to do, lifts that will target problem areas or just supplement the core lifts. If you lack time, just do your core lifts.

When lifting weights always keep body balance in mind. This will prevent injury and provide good body symmetry and aesthetic appeal. You do want to look better, right? Whatever you do for the top, do for the bottom, and whatever you do for the front, do for the back. This is a really important principle as it will prevent most injuries and get you balanced.[39] If you do three sets of ten repetitions (reps) for your chest, maybe a bench press movement, do three sets of ten reps with the opposing muscle group, your upper back. Do some type of rowing movement. (See wave4life.com for videos of all these movements) A repetition is one full movement of an exercise. If you are doing jumping jacks, it is one jumping jack, if you are doing push-ups, it is one push-up, etc. Here's an example of a balanced workout for your upper body:

1. Two sets of 20 reps for your shoulders, maybe shoulder press
2. Two sets of 20 reps for your latissimus dorsi (lats), the back muscles under your arms, maybe do pull-downs or pull-ups.
3. Two sets of 20 reps for your chest, maybe bench press or push-ups
4. Two sets of 20 reps for your upper back, maybe do rows

1 & 2 go together, and 3 & 4 go together; these are opposing muscle group exercises. If you want to figure out what the opposing muscle group is, or what a good exercise might be to exercise your opposing muscle group, just think *push and pull.* Shoulder press (military press) is the pushing movement, and lat pull-downs (or pull-ups) is the opposite pulling movement. Bench press (or push-ups) is the pushing movement, and rowing is the opposite pulling movement.

How many injuries could have been avoided in the weight room or on the athletic field if everyone just followed this simple principle of body balance? Millions. A good athletic trainer in rehabilitation (rehab) will check for imbalance, if one side of the opposing muscle group is proportionately out of balance.[40] If it is, they will have you strengthen the weak link. This is what you can do: If one part of your body is significantly weaker than the other, it is good to even them out. Some opposing muscle groups are supposed to be stronger

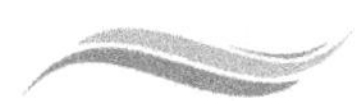

because there is more muscle there. For instance, your biceps (the front part of your arm) have two muscles, hence the word bi, and your triceps (the back of your arm) have three muscles, hence the word tri. Which do you think should be stronger? Your triceps because there is more muscle there. If you notice a significant difference in your strength levels between opposing muscle groups, and you train with other people and notice they do not have that same difference, it is probably your weakness. So, train that body part more, maybe even twice as much, until it evens out.

Another way to find your weaknesses is to look at your body in the mirror (mirror test). Is your body perfectly symmetrical? Is there anything really out of balance? Some people have a sway back, rounded shoulders, skinny chests...remember, you can change your body and even things out, it just takes a little work. That is why they call it a workout; everything worth anything in life takes work, right?

So, why would people not want to have good body balance and symmetry? Maybe the biggest reason is lack of knowledge. They think they were born this way and cannot do anything about it. Wrong. If you are fat, get the fat off. If you are weak or have an aesthetic flaw, make your weaknesses your strength. You might not be able to compete in the Olympic Games or be top in the nation in your age group, but you can balance things out. If you are slow, get faster. For those of you who are athletes, speed is the king of sport. If you want to be a good athlete, you will increase your speed. You can increase your speed through weight training, proper technique, sprinting (remember specificity), running hills and stairs, plyometrics, and stretching.

Other people are just plain lazy or do not care that much. Maybe they are married and figure, "I'm married, why should I worry about what I look like?" Ask the spouse how they feel about that. Even if your spouse really does not care, you should. It is just as important to your overall happiness and well-being to be fit, regardless of your marital status. Others are just too caught up in their daily lives to

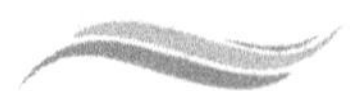

worry much about it. Balance is one of the great keys to living a healthy, happy, productive life. If your body is out of balance, so are you. We do function as a whole, and we are only as strong as our weakest link, so let's make our weaknesses our strengths.

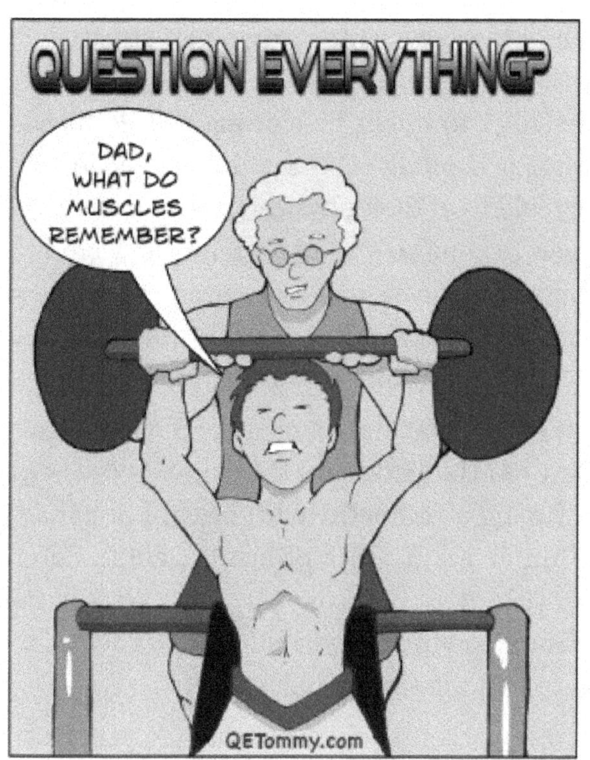

PRINCIPLE # 6 – Continually Change Your Workout

Avoid plateaus and physical and mental burnout

Your body will acclimate very quickly to whatever stresses you place on it, which is a wonderful thing. The problem is it will not continue to progress unless you place different stresses on it. In other words, continually change your workout so you will continue to progress.[41] There are masses of people all the time in the weight room and on the athletic field who never get any better. But they are out there every day working away at it all. *If you are not improving, you are doing something wrong!*

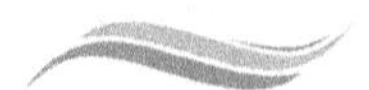

The only reason for not getting better at something you do every day, or often, is old age...even then you should be getting better at some things, especially those things which require more intellectual capacity and physical skill. You might be slowing a little physically, but you can make up for it mentally. Old age doesn't mean your late 20's or 30's. People should be at their physical peak in that age group. You can even be stronger in your 40's and 50's than you were in your 20's and 30's.[42] Your body might be a little more prone to injury, you might not recover as quickly, and you might have to work a bit harder, but you can probably out-do your former self even at these "older" ages.

There are some great stories of some amazing feats at relatively older ages. Dr. Fred Hatfield broke the world record at 42 years young in the squat. He did a competitive lift of 1014 pounds.[43] Nolan Ryan pitched a no hitter at 44 years of age.[44] George Foreman won the World Boxing Title at 45 years of age.[45] Tom Watson tied for the win at a major championship at 59 years of age.[46] The list goes on and on of what's possible in the second half of life.

Change your workouts so you continue to progress. Change it up every single month by doing something different. If it is weights you are doing, do more sets, less repetitions one month, do less sets more repetitions the next. Play basketball for 45 minutes one month, then next month drop it down to 20 minutes and go all out the whole time. Walk up and down the stairs five times a day one month, and ten times a day the next. Walk one mile a day one month, then two miles a day the next. Then maybe add in some stairs the next month.

Now, let's talk about cycling your workouts yearly.[47] Maybe your first three months you lay an aerobic base so there is a certain level of aerobic conditioning. Then the next three months you add in more strength training to establish more size, speed, and strength. Then the next three months you focus in on your objective and get very specific in your workouts, laying the foundation for the accomplishment of your objective. Then during the last three months you accomplish

your objective with very intense and specific workouts. Then you start all over the next year with a bigger goal and begin again with an aerobic base.

"Cycling is about a gradual build-up of intensity to a personal best, then starting all over with easy workouts...Cycling is the ultimate formula of strength which succeeds where other methods, often a lot more complicated, fail. Do yourself a favor and jump on the bandwagon with the world's strongest people. You will gain beyond your wildest dreams. You will suffer fewer, if any, injuries."

—Pavel Tsatsouline

Russian Strength Training Secrets for Every American

A good goal when working out in the weight room is to get your body sore every time you work out.[48] Not the kind of sore where it hurts to walk (as you get in shape you will get over this soon). The kind of sore where you can tell you pushed your body in ways it was not used to being pushed. You played baseball and stretched that double into a triple with a little extra effort, and you feel it in your hammies (hamstrings) the next day. You had your heart rate up close to your max heart rate in your walk this morning up that hill and you feel it in your lungs. You were breathing deeper than normal. You added a new stomach exercise to your workout yesterday, and you feel it in your abs (abdominals) today. If you enjoy the feeling push yourself to get a little sore. If it will scare you off from working out, do not do it. Some people love to get sore, and they don't mind a little pain. It lets them know they did something good. Other people have a very low tolerance for pain and absolutely hate being sore, even to the smallest degree. You will have to choose for yourself. You might start off not liking the pain but eventually thrive on it. Your pain tolerance will definitely rise as you push your body and get in shape.

When talking about pain, please be sure that you are not feeling the bad pain. There is good pain and bad pain. Bad pain will cause injury, so if you feel it, back off. It is usually sharp pain that lets you

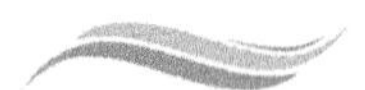

know you injured something or will injure something if you continue. Good pain is not sharp pain. It might hurt because you are pushing so hard, and you might be sore (more good pain) the next day, but you will not get injured. Be careful.

In your yearly cycle, remember to be careful with anything you do that is new, take it easy the first month. Your muscles have memory, which means they remember the training you have put into them in the past.[49] They will respond very quickly and bounce back to their original form. Tendons and ligaments do not have memory, so if you try to do what you have done in the past, without working into it, you will injure yourself.[50]

Many times, when people start something new that they have not done for a period of time they push themselves too hard. You might have been this strong a couple months ago, or a couple years ago, or could do it before, so your mind says you can do it, so do your muscles, but the tendons and ligaments cannot handle it. *Take it easy the first month!*

You also need to take time to stretch if you do not want to pull a muscle, and so your range of motion (ROM) increases. Flexibility should increase with age, by the way. Many people spend so much time increasing their strength but spend little or no time working on their flexibility. You will never notice the full benefits of your strength training if you do not increase your flexibility and range of motion.[51] Many times the added strength will actually decrease flexibility and the result will be a slower, less powerful, more prone to injury athlete or individual, not a better one. If you do pull a muscle, it will take you about 4-6 weeks to bounce back, maybe longer if it is a really bad pull. If you are an athlete in the middle of a season, this can wipe out a whole year. And if you are just getting started on an exercise program, this is another 4-6 weeks away from activity. Chances are if you are not in the habit of exercise, you will not come back for a lot longer than that. It makes sense to take a few minutes to stretch every day.

The best time to stretch to increase flexibility is after your workout, when your muscles are warmed up and loose.[52] Your muscles are like rubber bands. Is a cold rubber band easier to stretch or a warm one? Which one will stretch farther without breaking? Your muscles are no different. If you really want to increase your range of motion do partner stretches but be careful. You can injure the other person if you are not careful. Review some good stretches to use online.

If you are starting a strength-training program in the gym and have been away for a while, or even if it is a new exercise, stay in the 10 to 20 repetition range your first month, and *never, never, never train to failure.* Training to failure is training until you cannot do another repetition...stop a rep or two before failure. If you are doing a sport or activity and start feeling like you might get injured if you continue, or are too tired to continue, stop. If you are walking and feel like you cannot go another step, stop. Do not push it because you will get injured. The strongest athletes in the world do not train to failure, why would you?[53] Especially when just starting back up again. People ask all the time, how much weight should I use? The basic rule is never go below 10 repetitions your first month with any new exercise.[54] If the weight is so heavy that you cannot do at least 10 repetitions, or your activity is so intense that you cannot do it easily without pushing too hard, stop, do not continue, especially your first month.

Once you are past the first cycle of the year you can start to push yourself. The last cycle of the year should be your most intense, not necessarily with your strength training, but what it is you are training for. If you are in the middle of a football season build all your training up during the year for your season, so you can perform at your peak. Maybe you are in a marathon, gradually build your up miles and strength so when the day of the marathon comes around you are ready to give your best performance.

Keep yourself hungry. Not the food kind, the kind that makes your workout and playing fun. If your workout bores you, change it. Do something different. Unless everything you do bores you, then maybe you need an attitude adjustment. Change will keep you progressing and avoid mental and physical burnout.[55] Look forward to your workouts, and be excited with your progress. You are developing your whole self, BodyMindSpirit. This will give you inner peace and joy.

If your body is sore from a specific workout, do not do that same activity or exercise again. Rest your body or that specific body part. Do not work through soreness, your body will not progress like it should and you might get injured. The actual tearing of muscle fibers causes the soreness.[56] Your muscles need time and nutrition to rebuild, to come back stronger than before. If you do not wait until the soreness goes away, you are defeating the purpose. It is like being in a rowboat with one oar. You will go in circles.

If you are sore or injured, *work around pain, not through it*. Look at injury or soreness as an opportunity to focus and work on things you normally would not. Many people are so into their workout or activity that they push themselves to the point of injury, and then they still will not back off. If you have bad pain, or an injury, your body is telling you to back off, not to take some Ibuprofen, or get a cortisone shot, and continue. This philosophy is always amazing to behold. People take drugs to take the pain away so they can carry on. Your body knows when enough is enough. Have enough sense to listen!

All this does not mean that you should not do something every day. This means you should work another body part or do a different activity. Continually change your workout. Go get a massage. Massage is so under-rated here in the U.S. In Russia, and in many other countries in the world, massage is prescribed by doctors as therapy for whatever health problems that might exist due to stress and certain types of disease.[57] Americans tend to rely more on prescription drugs.

Learn how to enjoy life and everything it has to offer. Go for a bike ride in the mountains or take a walk on the beach. Take a car ride with a grandparent. Have a secluded candlelight dinner with

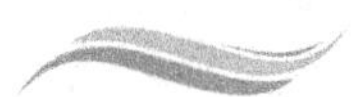

your sweetheart. Take time with a child to see things through four-year-old eyes. Focus on the beautiful things in life all around us, so you are not attracted to the sordid and corrupting influences that are also around us. Experience life fully, body, mind and spirit, and you will savor life and its sweet experiences. Of course, there is always the bitter, to make the sweet possible. You are in control, your life can be heaven or hell, it is up to you. Getting fit and enjoying the benefits can be pretty heavenly, I assure you.

QUESTION EVERYTHING?
LANI,
IF ELEPHANTS SIT WHERE
THEY WANT HOW DO YOU
TRAIN THEM?
QETommy.com

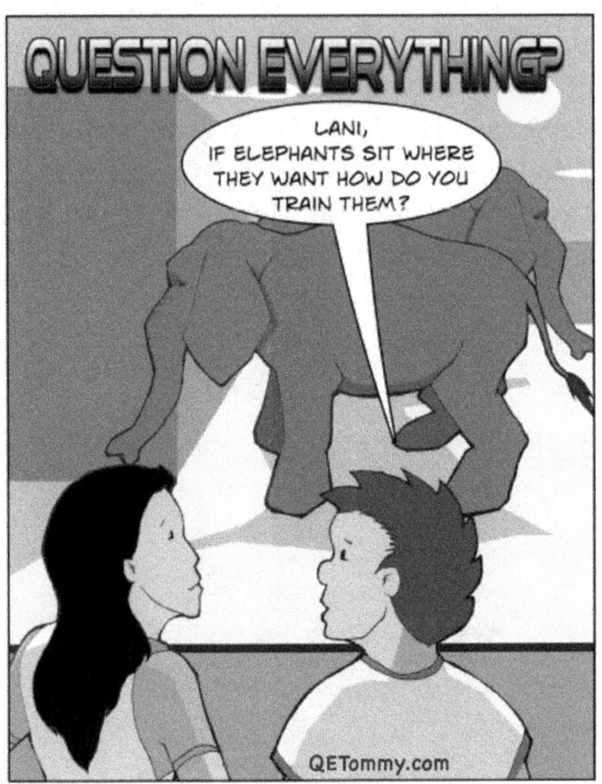

PRINCIPLE # 7 – Use A Bodymindspirit Approach To Your Fitness

Anything less and you go in circles

What good is it to be physically fit and neglect your mind or spirit? All three entities, BodyMindSpirit, function together and make you who you are. You are only as strong as your weakest link. When one part of you is underdeveloped, the other parts suffer, and you will never live up to your amazing potential, which is limitless.

Some people view the body as something that holds us back from achieving our true potential. Our bodies are sacred and a vital

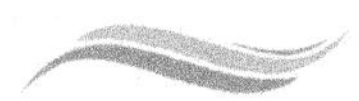

component to our progression.[58] Our mind and spirit direct our bodies, not the other way around.

If we eat properly, exercise, and avoid harmful substances, our bodies will be strong and vibrant. When we live a healthy lifestyle, we will avoid disease and make it much easier to have healthy minds and spirits.

Likewise, our minds are fertile soils. If we desire to be positive, we must take positive things into our minds. If we desire to be inspirational, we must feed our minds with inspiring thoughts. If we desire to be good and loving, we must expose our minds to good and loving things. The saying, "as a man thinketh in his heart so is he," is so true.

If we neglect our minds and do not challenge them daily, they will become weak. Just as our bodies and muscles become soft and diseased, so also will our minds if we do not use them. Is some mental illness caused by lack of mental exercise?[59] Yes. Mental illness can also be caused by an unhealthy body and/ or spirit. All three entities function as a whole. People try to separate them, but the reality is that each of us is a whole person.

What about our spirit? Without the spirit the body is useless, it is dead. Our spirits give light and life to our body.[60] Can we harm or destroy our spirits? We are eternal, BodyMindSpirit, we cannot destroy them, but we can harm them so they will not function properly. How do we harm the spirit? The same way we harm the body and mind, by improper maintenance, by forgetting our great potential and not living up to what we know to be true. When one part suffers, all parts suffer.

So, in our approach to health, let us consider our whole selves, BodyMindSpirit. Do not develop one part and neglect the others. Work on all three parts at the same time. Read good books, watch good movies, eat well, exercise, love people, do the right things, speak

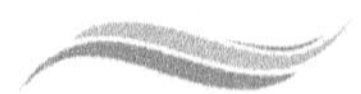

ill of no one, be the kind of person you know you can be. Herein lies true happiness, joy and peace. This is what most of us desire from life.

As you apply these 7 Principles of Exercise to your life, let WAVE help you. Sign up for some personal training, nutritional counseling, or coaching in the areas you need help the most, so you get these principles ingrained in you and they become part of your daily life. Live them and teach those you love to do the same. Your life will be blessed. Try some of the other WAVE products and services. Visit wave4life.com

QUESTION EVERYTHING?
GRANDMA, I WANT TO GAIN WEIGHT AND YOU WANT TO LOSE IT?
QETommy.com

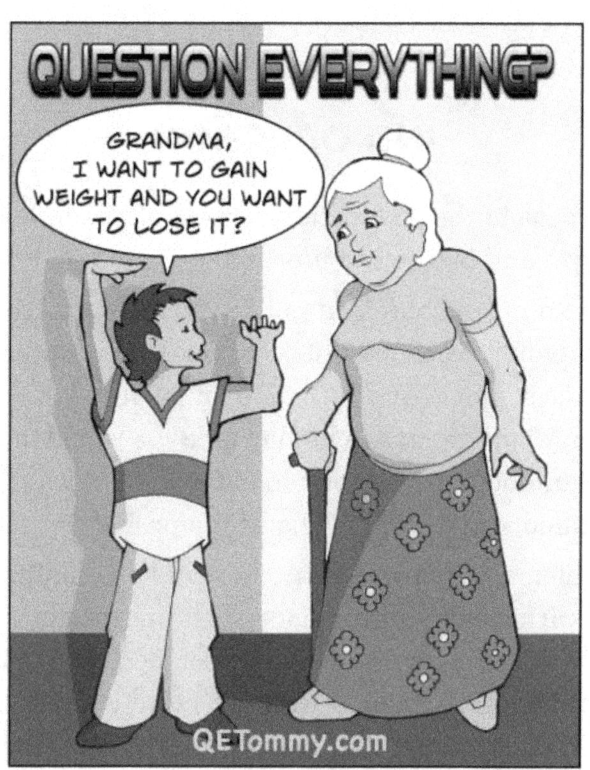

7 PRINCIPLES OF NUTRITION

"The number of overweight children between the ages of 6 and 11 has more than doubled since the late 1970's. According to surveys conducted by the Center for Health and Health Care in Schools and the National Association for Sport and Physical Education, parents support efforts by schools to strengthen exercise and nutrition programs to help halt the progression of childhood obesity. More than 70 percent of parents believe that physical education should be part of the school curriculum; that PE helps children perform better in the classroom; and that nutrition education should be included in the curriculum. Similar numbers of parents believe parents and schools should work together to plan school meals."

—American Dietetic Association

INTRODUCTION

The purpose of the 7 Nutritional Principles is to help you live a healthy, happy, and productive life.

There is so much confusion out in the marketplace...Should we lower the amount of carbohydrates? Should we eat bread and fruit? Should we take supplements? What about meat & dairy? With all the information available to us as a human race you would think we would be able to figure out what is good to eat and what isn't. It cannot be that complicated, can it? Then, what is the problem?

The problems are many: Vanity, false and misleading advertising, evil and conspiring men, convenience, gluttony, the quick fix, our fast-paced society, ignorance, pride, loss of perspective, biased research, corporate and political leaders who are more concerned with their own selfish interests rather than the common good of the people...the list goes on and on.

What can be done about it? The best thing to do is teach people true and correct principles, teach them how to live a healthy, happy, and productive life for themselves, which is the purpose of this book.[61] Why is teaching correct principles so effective? As people become more knowledgeable about truth, they naturally gravitate toward practices that really work. Once they try practices that really work, they become converted, they know for themselves that the underlying principle is true or correct. Thus, they are much more likely to follow the principle and live a healthier, happier life. The truth sets us free.[62]

What are ways we can determine if the principles we learn are true or correct? Certain things work and others don't. We can learn from those who have been down the path of experience. Another

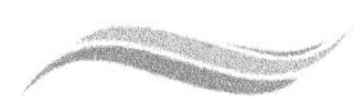

is ***current research***, without all the hype and money for slanted results; research for the sake of truth.[63] We should respect our modern world and all the information that is available to us as a human race. Information in our society is said to be doubling every few years, which is amazing, but let us be wise and discern the truth of this information. Otherwise, we can be forever learning and never come to a knowledge of the truth. We have seen this in so many generations before us. Often times in the area of nutrition; what is supported one day is not the next. If truth is really our objective, then we must seek it and hold true to it once we find it.

A third way to determine if something we learn is true is through ***revelation from God***.[64] This method will require personal study, prayer, and faith in sources like the scriptures, other inspired sources of truth, or personal belief in others who have pursued this path. Another way of determining if something is true is ***an appeal to logic***; some things just make perfect sense.[65]

This book teaches correct principles using all the above methods. It is founded on a search for true and correct principles. If you know of new research or find ideas you think could be better said, please send your comments to Tom at QETommy@icloud.com. Your suggestions will be taken seriously, as we are committed to continued searching and learning.

Remember that medical science is heavily based upon theory. Dr. L Jay Silvester, a 7-Time World Record holder in the discus and physical education professor, said it this way, "When it is said and done we really only understand about 10% of what goes on in our bodies, the rest is speculation."[66] A prestigious British medical journal in 1991 said, "*less than 15%* of all medical treatments given by doctors are based on sound scientific evidence because *less than 1%* of all articles in medical literature are scientifically sound."[67] You might say to yourself, if this is true, how can you write down 7 Principles that you say are true or correct? For the reasons listed above.

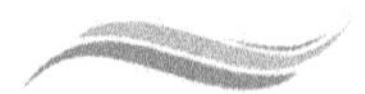

What about our most prized possessions, our children? The best thing you can do for your children is to be a good example because children ultimately imitate their parents. If our world is ever going to be a better place it will be through parents doing a better job raising their children.

"Train up a child in the way he should go:
and when he is old, he will not depart from it."

Proverbs 22:6

QUESTION EVERYTHING?
GRANDMA,
HOW COME WE SPEND THE
MOST ON HEALTH CARE BUT
RANK SO LOW IN THE
HEALTHIEST COUNTRIES?
QETommy.com

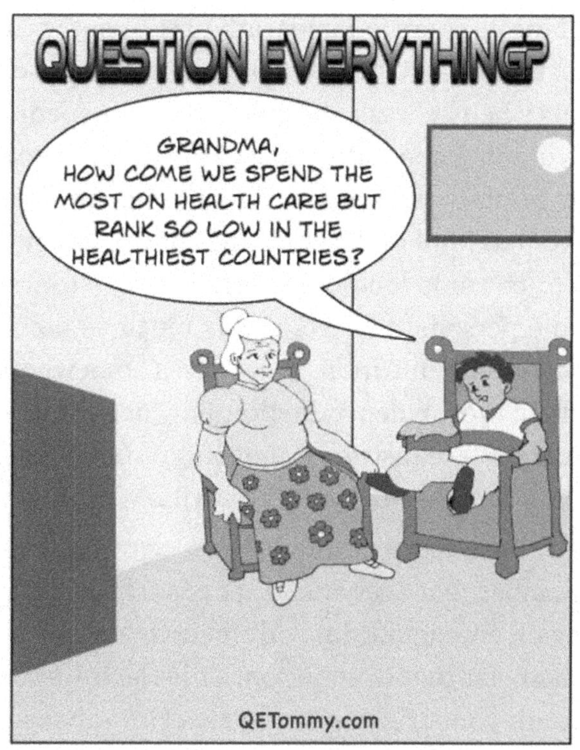

PRINCIPLE #1
Healthy Nutrition Is The Key To Good Health

"The best medicine is food"

—Hippocrates – Father of medicine

Healthy nutrition is the key to good health.[68] Dieting is a national preoccupation, but in this book, dieting is a *dirty* word. If you diet (starve yourself) you will eventually get fatter; it is a known fact.[69] Sumo wrestlers know this, and this is how they put their weight on. They skip breakfast, eat lunch after they train, take a 4-hour nap, then eat dinner right before they go to bed.[70] If great health is your goal, focus on *good nutrition,* not that dirty 4 letter word.

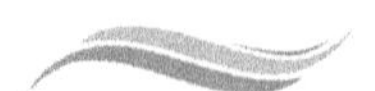

Another misconception many people have is; I'll exercise so I can eat anything I want. There is some truth to this, but with most people at least 50% of fat loss is related to nutrition not exercise.[71] If you are a Michael Phelps when he was in his 20's, where he spent 5 hours a day in the pool swimming about 800 laps of the pool, you can eat 12,000 calories a day of pretty much anything and not get fat. But most of us do not have that kind of desire or the time to spend working out. So there has to be some kind of balance between exercise and good nutrition. Some personal trainers say as much as *90%* of fat loss is directly related to our nutrition. Maybe it is somewhere in between those 2 numbers (70%), depending on how active we are? As these nutrition principles are discussed, hopefully you will come to better understand how important healthy nutrition is to your body and overall health and wellness.

Just remember that everyone responds a little differently. Some people never gain any significant body fat no matter what they do. But it is not just body fat that is important, it is the inward health of our bodies. What are your triglyceride levels? How about the good and bad cholesterol levels? Is there plaque build-up in your arteries? How many free radicals are flowing through your body? What are your antioxidant levels? What is your body's pH? Someone might have a really fast metabolism, have very low body fat, and look really healthy on the outside, but have plaque all over their arteries and suddenly drop dead of a heart attack, get Type II diabetes, osteoporosis, or cancer at an early age. Let's also consider our minds and spirits, our whole selves. Sooner or later bad habits catch up to people. It's the old saying, "you can pay me now or pay me later." It takes time and energy to take proper care of ourselves, BodyMindSpirit, but the benefits far outweigh the effort needed for proper maintenance. An ounce of prevention really is worth a pound of cure.[72]

What good is it to have an extra hour a day, the time it takes to exercise and make proper food choices, yet, not sleep well, feel tired,

stressed, sluggish and irritable, and die an early death? Not only do many people die early deaths, their *quality of life* the last few years of their life is terrible. They live far below their potential. Go to a nursing home some time to see what your destiny is like if you don't live a healthy life. It is definitely the exception that people who have lived healthy lives are in nursing homes. Most there have a very low quality of life. This low quality of life and all the problems associated with it costs Americans $billions every year that could have been saved by helping people live healthier lifestyles throughout their lives.[73]

"We spent over a $1 Trillion dollars on healthcare in 1997. In fact, the cost of our heath is spiraling so far out of control that the Health Care Financing Administration predicts that our system will cost $16 Trillion dollars by 2030."

—T. Colin Campbell – *The China Study*

According to the World Health Organization America spends more money on health care than any other country in the world, yet we rank only 37th in the health of our citizens.[74] The 2008 CIA Factbook says Americans rank 47th in the world in longevity, and total health care expenditures are more than $2 Trillion per year, or $6,697 per person.[75] This is more than double of any other country.[76] The Altarum Institute says that in 2008 only 8% of our health care money was spent on prevention, while the remaining 92% was spent on trying to fix the problems once they exist.[77] Cancer has gone from 1/33 in the early 1900's to more than 1/3 today.[78] Why is all this happening? What can be done?

In 2009 America spent over *$500 Billion* just on treating heart disease and stroke alone.[79] The average by-pass heart operation is well over $50,000 dollars.[80] This disease (our #1 killer) is preventable. Heart disease isn't something we catch; we do it to ourselves. It is usually developed through an unhealthy lifestyle. If everyone in America ate as much food as they wanted, but it consisted of less

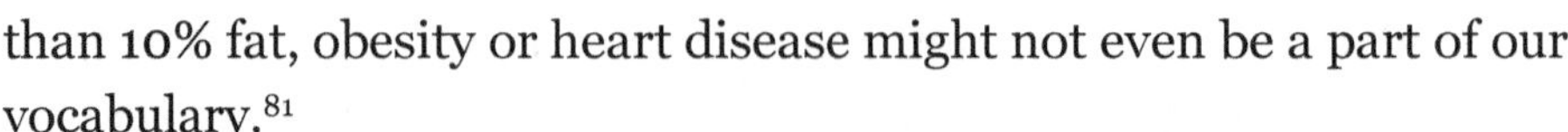

than 10% fat, obesity or heart disease might not even be a part of our vocabulary.[81]

How about diabetes? Type II (mature onset) diabetes is one of the most easily reversible diseases there is, through exercise and good nutrition, yet we spent over $100 Billion dollars on it in 2009.[82]

We must make a shift to more of a *preventative approach* in health care if we ever hope to truly solve our crisis. Countries like France and Japan focus much more of their attention on prevention.[83]

"In the 1970s, Finland had the world's highest incidence of deaths from heart disease. Not anymore. A public health campaign to educate people about diet, exercise, and the dangers of smoking helped slash heart disease deaths in the working-age population by 80 percent over the past three decades and added nearly ten years to the average Finn's life."

—Joe Kita[84]

We can and must make this shift – a shift that will help both America and the individual.

If people would change their lifestyles, Americans would not have most of the debilitating diseases we face as a nation. There is undeniable medical proof that most of the diseases we face as a nation are reversible and preventable. Read the New York Times best-selling book, *Dr. Dean Ornish's Program for Reversing Heart Disease: The Only Scientifically Proven System for Reversing Heart Disease Without Drugs or Surgery*. His statements are backed by undeniable research, and *thousands* of physicians across the country follow his program with their patients.[85] This is a must read because Americans have a 1 in 2 chance of developing this terrible disease; living a healthy lifestyle is your greatest strategy for preventing heart disease.

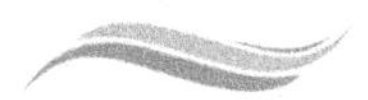

Tom's Training Client

In a personal training session a few years back in New York City I asked a personal training client of mine what he did for a living. He said, "I'm embarrassed to tell you." After I asked why, he said, "Because I work for an insurance company, and approximately 80% of what we spend on healthcare is *thrown* at the last 2 years of life."[86]

Is this absolutely insanity? People will do anything for loved ones when they are dying, but what about their quality of life when they are still living? Why not take some of this health care money and spend it on teaching people about good nutrition, how to *prevent* disease before it happens? Why not help share books like this one, and support companies like WAVE, that are educating the public on how to prevent disease before it happens? If we do this on a national scale this would save America billions of dollars every year on health care, and we would be a much healthier and happier people.[87]

Why so much talk about prevention when the discussion is supposed to be about nutrition? Because nutrition is prevention; and prevention is nutrition.

"Hippocrates, who lived from 460 to 377 BC, was known as the father of medicine. Orthodox doctors who take the Hippocratic Oath, but depend on man-made and therefore unnatural chemical medicines, should note that Hippocrates believed that 'the body has a tendency to naturally heal itself' and that 'food is the best medicine, and the best foods are the best medicines.'"

—Calcium Factor - Barefoot & Dr. Reich[88]

How did we get so far away from this common-sense approach to healthcare?

It's always unsettling to see all the hype about healthcare, and all the billions of dollars allocated to curing disease, with little or *no mention of prevention.* Over 90% of the money we spend on healthcare in America is spent on curative medicine, and less than

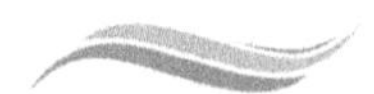

10% is spent on preventative medicine.[89] Yes, prescription drugs are important, and Medicare and Medicaid need to be there for our seniors and those in poverty, but if in America we did a better job of educating kids and parents, teaching them *how* to prevent disease, then most won't need prescription drugs, or need to spend a lot of time in the hospital when they get older.

How do we take control of our health and become healthier? The Mind Section talks extensively about life planning, but let's also talk a bit here about having goals. Don't just wander through life aimlessly. If it is decreased body fat you are after, then set a goal within a specific time frame. Write it down. It makes you more committed.

The majority of successful people write down exactly what they want to accomplish.[90] And if some successful people do not write down their goals they do not really need to. Why? Because their goals are so ingrained in their hearts and minds that they work hard every day to make their goals reality.

Maybe this year your goal is to run in a marathon, get your body fat below 15%, compete in a natural bodybuilding competition, or maybe you just want to be healthy enough to walk without assistance, or go for a walk with your grandchildren - whatever it is, have a goal.

Many people do not want to have a goal, or do not want to write it down, because they fear failure.[91] They get down on themselves, or are afraid they might look foolish in front of their peers if they do not achieve their goal, so it's easier to just forget about it. Others fear success.[92] This might seem odd, but they fear what achieving their goals might do to their life, or the lives of those around them. It is just safer and easier to keep on doing what they have always done and stay within their comfort zone.

It is critical to assess your current position in order to be able to set realistic goals. If you have no idea what your body fat is, how can you set a goal to get to a certain point? You might already be there! You might want to throw the weight scale out the door by the way. It

doesn't mean much. The body mass index (BMI) is a good measure when applied to the entire population but may not be sensitive to individual anomalies. For instance, for a muscular person the body mass index score will be higher due to the muscle mass. It is easy to calculate your BMI using the Internet. The simple height and weight charts that many physicians and health care professionals use are outdated.[93] These are averages, and you might not be average. You might have big, thick, dense bones, or you might have thin, light bones. You might have a lot of muscle mass on your body, or not much. The averages don't tell you the whole story. An accurate body fat measurement is a better test to measure both your health and appearance.[94] Buy a body fat scale or, if possible, go to a local college and get your body fat measured. Also complete the Fitness Assessment in the Appendix. It is very important to have a *true starting point*, and don't cheat. Stay motivated and work toward your goal. If you know where you are, you will get excited upon periodic testing because you will see progress and the possibility of continual improvement.

There is another great device called, a BioPhotonic Scanner, that came out in 2004 which measures your antioxidant levels.[95] This gives you quantifiable evidence about how many antioxidants are flowing through your body. The BioPhotonic Scanner is highly motivational for choosing good nutrition. The only problem is it is not available yet in the general market except through a network marketing company called Pharmanex. Basically, you have to go to one of their distributors, or their company headquarters, to get measured. They have an exclusive on the device. See if there is a distributor near you and get measured. Just look them up on the web. This device is amazing. It takes the measurement on the palm of your hand, and it measures about 6 weeks back, so it doesn't do any good to eat really well or take a bunch of antioxidants right before you go in to get measured. The device is very accurate.[96] Average scores range from about 10,000

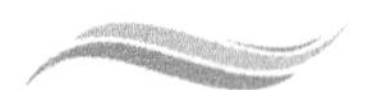

– 15,000. Some vegetarians, raw foodists, and interestingly enough people who eat a lot of berries (blackberries, blueberries, raspberries, strawberries, etc.), foods that are high in their Orac Value (quantity of antioxidants), have been measured as high as 80,000 – 100,000. Supplementation also helps.

Whatever you are measuring, keep in mind that testing methods are critical.[97] It is very frustrating for both the trainer and client when improvement is noticed yet an inaccurate test does not represent the progress made. When you are testing, use the most accurate methods possible. Maybe you live near a college or university where you can get your body fat measured with a $50,000 device for a nominal $15 fee.[98] Maybe you want to see if you can hit the baseball farther since you have been strength training. Make sure you use the same kind of balls each time, and use the same bat with the same speed pitch, in the same weather so it will be an accurate comparison. Or maybe you are measuring your time in the 100-yard dash, or how long it takes you to walk 2 miles. Measure it at the same track, with the same shoes, the same time of day and the same food intake, the same person timing you, and start the clock the same way (on your move). You get the picture.

Remember that *healthy nutrition* is the key to good physical health. This section talks extensively about what is good and bad to put into your body. In short if you center your nutrition around fruits, vegetables, and whole grains, including legumes, nuts and seeds, you will likely be very healthy.[99] Once you become more educated and gain a better idea of what you want to eat, then set some realistic goals and strive to be your best self. You will be amazed by your progress and how good you feel. There is always room for improvement.

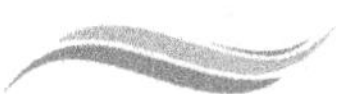

NOTE: If you are not close to a college or university with a good body fat measuring device, you can buy a Tanita Body Fat scale.[100] You can buy it at, wave4life.com, and it will be drop shipped to your doorstep. Or visit your local sporting goods store; they should have one. If you are an athletic person (with a lot of muscle on your body), buy one that has an athlete mode which is a little more expensive; if you are athletic and get the regular one it will measure you high. The Tanita Body Fat scale is an easy way to get your body fat, and it is the most consistent method available to most people. Though the Tanita Scale is not the most accurate method (hydrostatic weighing is one of the most accurate methods), it should be fairly consistent. *Consistency* of measurement is the most important factor since we are most interested in measuring *improvement*.

QUESTION EVERYTHING?
MOM,
DO DIETS MAKE
PEOPLE FATTER?
QETommy.com

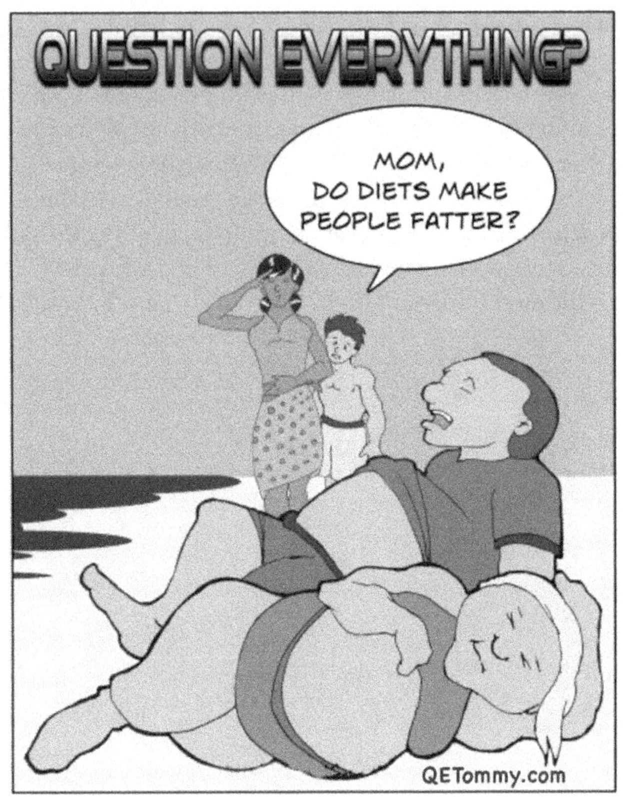

PRINCIPLE #2
Find Your Healthy Body Fat Level

You are in control

There are several things you can do to have a healthy percentage of body fat. Your nutrition is a key factor; what you eat, how often you eat, how much, if you drink enough water, if you supplement, and of course exercise. For more information about exercise see the Exercise Section, just know the time you do it, how often you do it, and what you do are key factors in having healthy body fat levels.

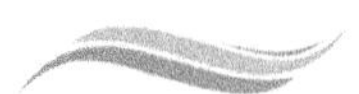

Eat *4-6 meals daily*.[101] Is this too much you might ask yourself? No. C*onstant* nourishment is a key factor in maintaining consistent energy levels, a healthy metabolism, and healthy body fat levels.[102] After you eat your food is broken down and enters your bloodstream to supply your body with needed nutrients. Your blood sugar (energy) levels will be higher after you eat and your food is digested. When you haven't eaten for long periods of time, like in the morning after you wake up, your blood sugar levels will be low. If you eat many (4-6) small meals throughout the day your blood sugar levels will remain constant, thus insuring the best possible nutrition to your body. It will also provide consistently high energy, a fast metabolism, and optimal mood levels throughout the day.[103]

Children naturally eat like this; they like to eat small meals often. Yet parents often get mad at their kids for wanting to eat so regularly. They are *teaching us* how to take proper care of our bodies and we are getting mad at them? Adults can be pretty dumb sometimes. The sad part is when kids grow up being forced to eat fewer and larger meals; it may make them gain weight.

The toughest part about personal training is that habits are formed over a lifetime. Many times, even though people do change their bad habits they go back to their old habits over time. This is why WAVE is so effective! We teach people correct principles that work, and then there is an immediate support system in place for people to change their lives. Hire a coach (Personal Trainer, Registered Dietician, etc.) to help you change your bad habits. Then rehire them, or get on a maintenance program, whenever you feel yourself slipping, or just need that extra boost of support. Of course, prayer will always be a great source of strength and can be a consistent part of your healthy living.[104]

Whenever you eat, your body revs up to digest and use the food you just consumed. This causes your metabolism to speed up. Every time you eat it raises your metabolism.[105] When you raise

your metabolism it is easier to burn fat off your body. This is one of the hardest lessons for women to learn because so many have been taught their whole lives to starve themselves to lose weight. When you starve yourself, or take long periods between meals, your metabolism slows down because your body recognizes a starvation situation, which is unhealthy.[106] Your body has to have fuel, and if it doesn't get what it needs it will store food as fat, so it has fuel for continued use. Your fat stores act as stored energy for your body.[107] Your body goes to them when the blood sugar levels get low. What would happen if you starved yourself and there was no body fat? Your body would cannibalize itself then you would die. This is why your body needs constant nourishment, so your body doesn't go into survival mode and store a bunch of body fat. You also will have consistent blood sugar levels to feel bright and alive. Constant blood sugar levels mean constant energy and more consistent mood levels.

People are starting to accept this philosophy, but the *diet* (4 letter word, remember?) *revolution* has been around for centuries, and has taught people to starve themselves (lower their caloric intake) to lose weight.[108] Starvation diets will probably always be around because many people want the *quick fix*; they want to get skinny for that high school reunion, that big date, grand ball, or the summer, but do not want to do what it takes to live healthy lives. Starvation dieting works, but the sad reality is that people probably lose more muscle than fat and will end up gaining all their weight back plus more. Why? Because their metabolism slows down whenever they starve themselves, and they lose muscle, both of which burn fat. People lose muscle when they diet because muscle needs nutrition to survive. Poor nutrition may cause a loss of muscle, and muscle does not come back easily.

"Diet books routinely top the best seller lists, and new plans come out seemingly every day. Do they work? Will any of them be right for you? If you are considering one or more popular diet or exercise plans, you owe it to yourself and your health to make sure

their claims are valid. Ask yourself: Does the diet plan promise a quick fix? Encourage or require you to stop eating certain foods, food groups or products? Rely on a single study as the basis for its recommendations? Contradict recommendations of reputable health organizations? Identify good and bad foods? Just sound too good to be true? If you answered yes to any of these questions, keep looking – for a plan that is backed by solid science, lets you keep eating your favorite foods, and allows for flexibility."

—American Dietetic Association

In the early 90's a 20-year study was completed by the U.S. Government on the success rate of some of the major diet centers across the nation.[109] They found a *99.8% failure rate*. Nearly 100% of the time these people who paid good money to lose weight gained all their weight back plus more. This is criminal. This isn't weight loss; they should be called weight gain centers. ☺ Since this study came out many of these diet centers have changed their programs, but there is still the desire to keep people coming back or keep them buying "their" food. WAVE does not have any diets. If anything, you will likely be encouraged to eat more food, not less. WAVE teaches people about healthy nutrition! Please remove that dirty word (diet) from your vocabulary, and replace it with the positive one, *healthy nutrition*. Please forget about all the diets out there that you hear about, they do not work. All they do is slow down your metabolism and eventually make you fat.[110]

"Each diet lowers the metabolic rate more than the previous diet, and it takes longer each time for the metabolic rate to recover. Weight is gained more rapidly after each diet, and the same low-calorie diet becomes less and less effective at removing the weight from the dieter's body with each successive try."

—Dr. Marc Sorenson – National Institute of Fitness[111]

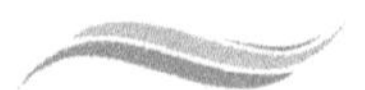

As most dieters are misinformed, where do they turn for truth? Many obese people actually eat less than skinny people. Is it their fault they are obese? No, it's because of the corrupt world we live in. Yes, many obese people do eat a lot of food, but how many have tried over and over to lose weight and finally givc up?

Does the *quantity* of food matter? Yes and No. How's that for a direct answer? If the *quality* is high enough, the quantity doesn't matter much (see Principle #4 - Eat High Density Foods).[112] It depends on the individual and the situation. Many people overeat for psychological reasons. Food is a kind of anti-depressant from pain. They turn to it whenever they feel bad about themselves, or bad about life. Others overeat to protect themselves from those who have abused them. They figure if they are obese their abusers will leave them alone. Others eat much more than needed because they have been very physically active in the past, and their bodies and minds are used to eating a lot of food. Others are lacking some critical nutrients from their nutrition and their bodies thus have tremendous cravings. People should eat regularly, *constant nourishment*, even if obese.[113] You will understand more of the reasons why as the discussion progresses. Generally, be more concerned with the *quality* than quantity of the food you consume.

Don't be slovenly and stuff yourself until you feel sick. Listen to your body; if you're hungry, eat, when you are full, stop. Let's add a caution here. Some people are rarely hungry because their bodies are so used to starvation, 1 or 2 meals a day, so their body no longer feels the hunger pains. The key is to turn your body into a *fat burning machine.*[114] If you do you will be ready to eat all the time. This is a good thing. Your body is always ready for food, and it will burn it off soon after you consume it. People like this usually have very low body fat because their metabolisms are so high. This is what we are after, and why *constant nourishment* is so important. Does this mean you should eat if you are not hungry? Yes. Do this

until you can condition your body to have regular meals. Turn your body into a fat burning machine by eating every 3-4 hours. That's 4-6 small meals per day, with one of those being a big meal *before* your workout.

Did you know that most anorexic people have over 30% body fat?[115] They look in the mirror and see the fat so they continue to starve themselves. Most people around them say, "you are not fat, you are skinny." Yes, they are skinny in clothes, but they are fat when they look in the mirror. Their bodies have gone into survival mode due to the lack of nutrition. They store fat very effectively, and most of their muscle has fallen off their body. It is a very sad situation. If they only understood correct principles of fat loss, they might not have any more desire to starve themselves. No doubt there would not be so many people starving themselves or throwing up after they eat trying to get skinny. This is a terrible problem in our colleges.[116] There is tremendous pressure on young women to be skinny. Many gorge themselves on the food and get rid of it afterward (bulimic), thinking they will be thin. Chances are most of these girls will become obese over time because they are living in such an unhealthy manner.

Our body has memory.[117] When people continue to do starvation dieting the body finally says, "OK, that's enough, you are continuing to starve me, and I never know when you are going to do it again, so I will permanently lower my metabolism and store a lot of body fat so you don't one day kill me off." This is why many obese people eat less than skinny people. Their metabolism rates are so low that they get fat just looking at food. The good part is we can get rid of our slow metabolism and speed it back up to normal. Isn't our body amazing? However, as Dr. Sorenson says, the more you have done this to your body, the more resistant it will be to change.

Your body needs *constant nourishment*. Keep your metabolism high. Take good supplements. Take healthy snacks with you throughout

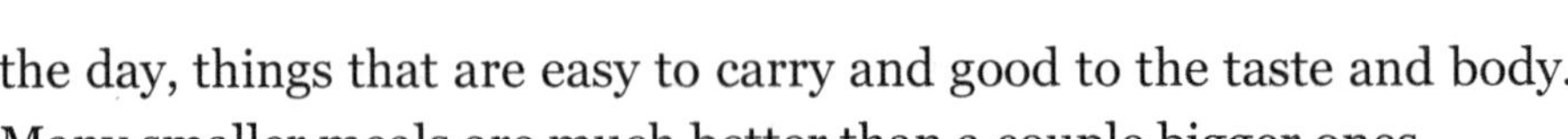

the day, things that are easy to carry and good to the taste and body. Many smaller meals are much better than a couple bigger ones.

A simple analogy is how we fuel our cars...do you go on a long trip then fill up your car with gas, or do you fill up your car with gas then go on the trip? This is a ridiculous question, right? Then why would we treat our bodies this way? The sad part is most people do. Something like 80% of what we consume as Americans is eaten after 7pm at night.[118] Which meal is typically the largest here in America? Dinner, right before we go to bed. People go to work, maybe skipping breakfast, or have white bread and coffee, work hard during the morning, then often eat an unhealthy lunch, or maybe even skip it. Work hard again in the afternoon (feeling terrible physically and mentally), then at the end of the day head home to a great dinner and gorge themselves on all the good food because they are famished. Then lie around watching TV and go to bed a couple hours later. Sound familiar anyone?

If you are going to go to sleep you do not need a lot of energy to do that, right? So, eat a smaller meal. If you are going to go workout in a couple hours, eat a large meal so you have the energy. The largest meal of the day should be *before* your exercise routine, not after. If you exercise at night, make dinner your biggest meal. If you exercise in the morning, get up early and eat a big breakfast.

Some people like to exercise on an empty stomach.[119] It is not good to exercise on an empty stomach, and if you think you do your best workouts on an empty stomach, think again. Your blood sugar is low because you have gone all night without nutrition. Food is your energy source; you are *running on empty*. A great performance will *always* be lacking.

It is true that you will likely burn more body fat on an empty stomach. This method is tried by many people to lose body fat, but it is a quick fix that will not work long term. When you go all night without eating your blood sugar is very low (low energy), and then when you

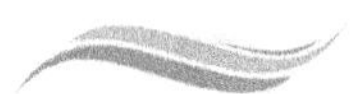

exercise your body needs energy. If there is not much blood sugar available where does your body go for energy? Your stored body fat. But there are a couple questions; does the lower performance offset the fat burning? In other words, you will not be able to perform as well in your workout if your blood sugar is low. Is this lower performance in your workout going to be better because you are using energy from your fat stores, or would it just be better to eat, have good blood sugar levels, work out harder, and thus affect your body more with a better workout? And how about your metabolism, does it lower because you are depriving your body? It makes sense that it would.

When is the best time for you to work out? As mentioned in the Fitness Section, when you are best fed and most rested. If you are only doing one workout a day it might make sense to work out in the afternoon or evening, after a great meal. Why? Because it might be tough for you to get up early enough in the morning to have a great breakfast, let your body digest the food, then workout, especially if you have kids. You might be able to get away with exercising on a full stomach if you walk or do something that is light. But if you are doing whole body exercises like squats, or running stairs, things that take a lot of physical energy and focus, it will not likely sit well (literally) with lots of food in your stomach. So maybe the afternoon or evening makes more sense? If you work hard during the day, you'll likely be tired at night, then a workout in the morning or during the day before you get too tired makes more sense.

The low carbohydrate (carb) diet is so prevalent in our society, let's talk a bit more about it here.[120] Some people prefer to do the no/ low carb thing after a certain time in the day. They do this because they are trying to burn more body fat. It works, but remember, low carbs = low energy.[121] If you are not doing anything really active at night you will not notice the energy drop as much. If people insist on going low carbs, which is not healthy, then do it at night. Don't cut out your carbs during the day unless you want to irritate everyone around

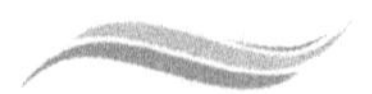

you. Why? Because you will be grouchy and irritable when your body lacks the nutrition it needs. If you insist on cutting the carbs, cut them out after a certain time in the afternoon or evening.

"Do you ever find yourself in the middle of a thought and suddenly it's gone? Or maybe in the middle of the afternoon your mind begins to wander? Your brain may be telling you something. Your brain needs fuel just like the rest of your body. Since your brain cannot store glucose, it needs a continuous source of fuel from foods. Start with a nutritious breakfast and continue with healthy meals and snacks through the day. Foods like blueberries, strawberries, prunes, and fatty fish show a positive benefit to short-term memory."

—American Dietetic Association

It's amazing that people do not listen to their bodies; they don't eat, or they pull all the carbs out of their nutrition, and then wonder why they have no energy. Our bodies have fats, proteins and carbohydrates to choose from for energy. The first thing our bodies go to for energy is ***carbohydrates***. It is easy for our bodies to break carbs down into glucose (our bodies needed energy source) ...then why would we pull carbs out of our nutrition? *It makes no sense.*[122] Why is the low-carb diet so popular? Probably because it can pull fat off quickly (with questionable long-term results), and because people can eat all the meat and fat they want, which appeals to many people. We live in a quick fix, gluttonous society.

The conversion of fat to energy takes much longer than carbohydrates to energy and is much harder for the body.[123] This is why you feel so sluggish and tired (low energy) on a low-carb diet. When you eat carbohydrates on the other hand you feel good (unless they are simple carbs), your body has an easy time processing them into energy. If carbs break down easily and give us immediately energy, it makes sense to eat them before periods of intense exercise, or when we need to be alert and attentive. If fats and proteins take

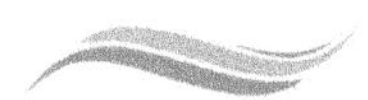

longer to break down, it makes sense they might be best to eat when we need extended energy or need to go longer periods of time without food. Maybe the best time to eat foods that break down slower is at dinner, when we go to sleep for 8 hours, and don't eat for 12 hours total. Remember, our bodies preferred energy source is *complex* carbohydrates. Complex carbs come from things like fruits, vegetables, and whole grains (including legumes). Simple carbs come from things like sugar, pop and pastries.

Never cut the complex carbs out of your nutrition. But for fat loss low carbs might be better than the low calories, because most low-carb diets suggest that you keep your calories up, so your body doesn't go into starvation mode, thus lowering your body's metabolism. Of course, it is always best to eat sensibly, centering our nutrition around food we all know is good for us on a daily basis; meals consisting of fruits, vegetables and whole grains (including nuts, seeds, and legumes).

We should be conscious of our carbohydrate/ protein/ fat ratios throughout the day. There have been many books written on this subject, The Zone (40-30-30) was a popular one (carbs being 40, fat and protein being 30 each).[124] Ratios more like 70/15/15, or 80/10/10 are healthy.[125] 80% carbs – mostly complex from fruits, vegetables & whole grains (w/ legumes, nuts & seeds); 10 % proteins – mostly from whole grains, beans, rice, nuts, vegetables and fruit; 10% fats - mostly from vegetables, nuts, and seeds.

This 80/10/10 nutrition program might seem contrary to what you have heard the last few years, and it might scare many people. People have been conditioned to think that carbs are bad. Simple carbs are bad, but complex carbs are good. Remember, fruits, vegetables, and whole grains are mostly carbohydrates. Everyone knows these foods are good for us. Carbohydrates are our bodies preferred energy source; our bodies have the easiest time converting carbohydrates into energy. It just isn't that complicated. It's simple and easy to

maintain healthy body fat levels, and have consistent energy, when you live by correct principles of fitness and nutrition.

You can easily drop your body fat levels if you up the protein in your nutrition. This high protein/ low fat method is probably the most popular method used amongst bodybuilders for lowering their body fat and getting ready for competition. Sometimes they will eat a 1:3 ratio of carbs to protein; something like 20/70/10, with their fat coming from things like lean fish, nuts, or flaxseed oil. Again, this method works. But the long-term health of eating this much meat or protein is highly questionable. Our bodies go into ketosis with too much protein, which is a sickly state. Plus, we will get dehydrated because it takes so much water to digest all the meat. Many people who eat like this look great, but they are not healthy, and it catches up to them. Eventually they will look old and sickly from abusing their bodies.

Check out the book by Dr. T. Colin Campbell entitled, *The China Study*. In it Dr. Campbell says that his research indicates that disease (heart disease, cancer, osteoporosis, etc.) kicks in anytime we eat more than about 5% animal protein.[126] So, the 10% protein suggest might be too much if it comes from animal sources, but we're OK since most of what is suggested comes from vegetables, fruit, whole grains, nuts and seeds. Too much meat is hard on our digestive system, especially the tougher meats, because it takes so many harsh chemicals and such a long time to break the meat down for digestion. It takes about 3 days or more (if our body is functioning properly) to digest meat through our long intestine.[127] We have the same type of intestine as the cow and horse, who are grass and grain feeding animals.

Please note that this book does not promote vegetarianism or being a vegan (no meat or dairy), but it does promote eating meat sparingly. The Bible says that meat is ordained for the use of man, and this book will never teach anything which is contrary to the teachings

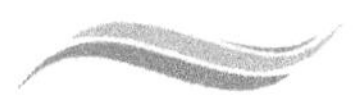

of the Bible.[128] Meat is something that is best viewed as a delicacy or treat, like dairy, not something to center our nutrition around.

Upping protein is not the only way to lower your body fat. There are many methods which are healthy that will help you including eating many smaller meals, and not eating big meals before you go to bed. Principle # 4 talks extensively about another common-sense method that will help you keep your body fat low, which is eating foods high on the Nutrient Density Chart. Principle #6 is also a great way to lower your body fat, by eating foods low on the Glycemic Index. Raw food also works, as do most vegan and vegetarian nutrition programs, as long as you avoid the simple carbs. Go to a vegan meeting some time, you will notice that most vegans have low body fat. These are *healthier* ways to drop your body fat.

Whenever you mention vegan or vegetarian living *protein* always pops up as a big concern. This concern is logical, but not valid, if we eat healthy. Our muscles are made up of 100% protein. Well, actually about 70% water, all the rest is protein. So, it makes sense that we need protein in our nutrition to give our muscles the necessary building blocks they need. We need protein at every meal. The question then becomes, how much do we really need?

Only 5-6% of our total calorie intake needs to come from protein in order to replace the protein we lose every day through body excretions.[129] A study in the American Journal of Clinical nutrition said we only need 2.5% of our total caloric intake from protein.[130] For the last 50 years the Government's RDA for protein is .8 grams per kilogram (1 kilogram = 2.2 pounds) of body weight, which is about 10% of our total caloric intake.[131] Many bodybuilders, on the other hand, say we need as much as 1 – 2 grams of protein per day per pound of body weight.[132] They say a 200-pound man would need about 200-400 grams of protein daily. This can amount to over 30% of total caloric intake coming from protein, which is 5-10 times more

than we really need. Many bodybuilders eat meat 4-7 times a day plus consume supplements that have 50-100 grams or more of protein at a time. This is very excessive and cannot be good for the body. It might help create big lean bodies, but it is really hard on the body to consume this much protein when it is in the form of meat or animal protein. Looks can often be *very* deceiving.

Consider that many vegetables and fruit are more than 10% protein. See online for a longer list, but here are a few. (Source is the U.S. Department of Agriculture):[133]

1. Spinach – 49% protein
2. Wheat germ – 31% protein
3. Cauliflower – 40% protein
4. Lentils – 29% protein
5. Wild Rice – 17% protein
6. Lemons – 16% protein
7. Honey Dew – 10% protein
8. Broad Bean – 31% protein
9. Tomatoes – 18% protein

You can see if you eat nutrition high in fresh fruits and vegetables you will be getting a high percentage of protein in every meal. Nuts and seeds are also very high in protein. So are whole grains. It is very clear that we *do not* need to eat meat, or have high quantities of animal protein, to get the protein that what we need in our nutrition.[134] There is *a lot* of controversy about all this. There is powerful lobby going on that most of us are not aware of, and we have been conditioned since the time we were children to eat lots of meat and dairy to "get our protein." Look around, it is everywhere, but the science behind the hype is lacking.

Read for yourself and come to your own conclusions. The book *The China Study* is a good source for credible information. *The New York Times* called it the "Grand Prix of epidemiology", with over

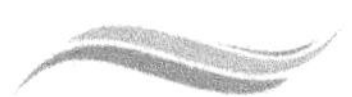

8,000 statistically significant associations between lifestyle, nutrition, and disease.[135] *Mega Health* by Dr. Marc Sorenson, the founder of the National Institute of Fitness, is also a great source, as are other books like, *Eat to Live*, by Dr. Joel Fuhrman, who is a practicing physician and has worked with over 10,000 patients, and Dr. Dean Ornish, who has a tremendous following of physicians across America...the list goes on and on, but here are four great authors on nutrition.

Most everyone in the world agrees that fruits, vegetables, whole grains, and legumes are good for us. A few people might preach against some of these in large quantities, but few, if any, would argue that we should not eat these things, which are mostly made up of carbohydrates. So why do so many American's think carbohydrates are of the devil? Maybe as you continue reading you will better understand.

What are the best sources of protein? Again, most often people say meat and dairy because they have so much protein in them, have all 20+ essential amino acids (the building blocks of protein) that our bodies need, are readily available in our society, very inexpensive (compared to the resources it took to create it), and are low in carbs. Also, much of our meat supply is very low in fat these days. So, it fits in with what many people are trying to accomplish, a big lean body.

Many say meat gives us all the amino acids we need, and that fruits, vegetables, and whole grains do not. Our bodies actually produce many of the amino acids (proteins) that our bodies need, so there are only about 8 essential amino acids that we need from our nutrition.[136] Most all fruits, vegetables, and whole grains *do* have all of these essential amino acids that meat does, but they do not have them in the same quantities.[137] Also, we used to think that we needed all our amino acids at every meal, but it has been found that our bodies can actually store amino acids (protein), so it really isn't important to get all the amino acids in one meal like we used to think.[138]

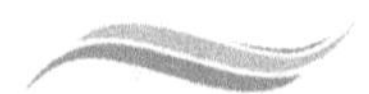

Again, please don't view these words as meat bashing, because this is not what is going on. Meat is ordained of man, it is a wonderful food, and a little bit of it is likely good for us. But it makes sense to eat meat sparingly and be very *thankful* for each piece we eat because it took the life of an animal, and so many of the earth's resources, to create it.

Did you know that if an animal is grain fed, it takes about *20 pounds* of grain to create one pound of meat?[139] How many people would the 20 pounds of grain feed versus that one pound of meat? You don't have to be too smart to figure that one out. 20 pounds of grain might feed 20 people for a day; one pound of meat might feed one person.

"The earth has enough for everyone's need,
but not enough for everyone's greed."

—Mahatma Gandhi

It is because of the greediness and gluttony of man that people go hungry. The other big problem with our meat supplies these days is unless you are getting the good stuff, organic meat, or some you've raised or hunted yourself, you are likely not getting what you think you are getting.

Become informed about our meat supplies. Find out what foods the animals were raised on. Some of the stories will make you sick; the steroids, growth hormone, chemicals, that they have put in the animals, and how they have treated the animals, and the things they feed them would literally turn your stomach. It is really sad to hear some of the conditions these animals are raised in.[140] Buy organic meat or hunt your own. Organic meat is generally grain-fed, steroid and growth hormone free, and the animals are free roaming, which means they give the animals some space to run around. But be careful even with organic meat because it is a relatively new field there are not as many laws associated with it.

Another thing to consider is how soft the meat is that you eat.

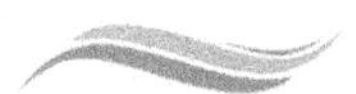

Doesn't it make sense that it takes a lot more digestive enzymes and harsh chemicals in your digestive tract to break down the tougher meats you eat? Eat more of the softer meats, things like fish vs. the tougher red meats like steak. But there is nothing like a great steak every once in a while, right? ☺ Never completely eliminate anything from your nutrition, enjoy your time at the table.

Be wise, listen to your body, and make sensible choices. Eat as close as possible to mother earth (nothing with a label on it), and things free of hormones, pesticides, and other chemicals and processing. You will never go wrong with fruits, vegetables, and whole grains, including legumes, nuts, and seeds, all in their purest form; these are the things that are best to center our nutrition around.

QUESTION EVERYTHING?
MOM, IF WE KNOW THE THINGS THAT CAUSE CANCER, WHY ARE WE STILL LOOKING FOR A CURE?
HOSPITAL
QETommy.com

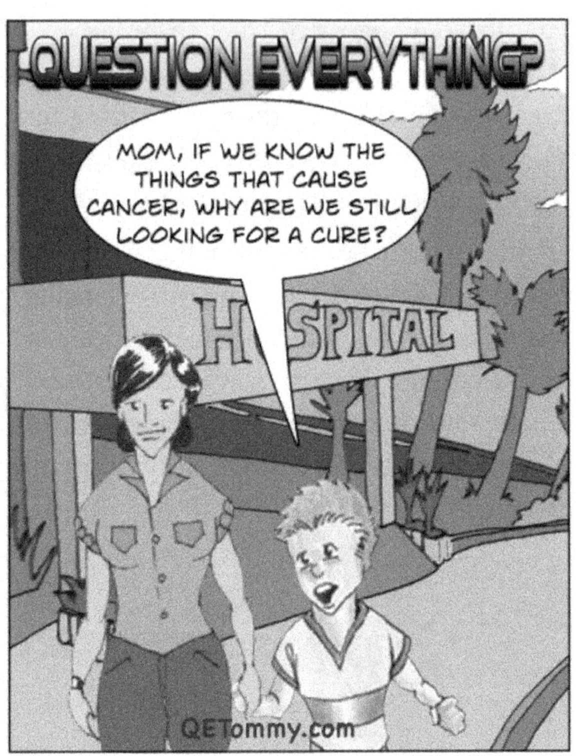

PRINCIPLE # 3
Free Radical /pH Balance Theories

*What If...*we already know the cause of cancer & how to cure it?

NOTE: Before we start, we would like to add some caution. Neither Tom Wright, wave international, nor any of it's officers, divisions, agents, employees, or independent contractors accept any responsibility for any advice given here. These are opinions only. you have the God-given right to treat yourself as you believe is best. Please be cautious and use wisdom and prayer to discern what is best.

These cautions need to be stated because here in America nobody but a physician can tell you how to cure any disease. But people need

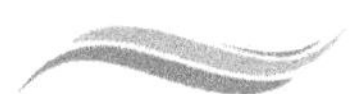

to know what is going on in the marketplace, understand wisdom of past and present, and know what God has said on the subject of staying healthy. If nothing else remember these words, *your body is the thing that will cure you*; give it the nutrition, rest, exercise, peaceful thoughts it needs, and it will heal itself.[141]

Hippocrates, a Greek physician who became known as the Father of Medicine, was regarded as the greatest physician of his time. He based his medical practice on observations and the study of the human body, rather than mysticism and superstitions of his time. He held the belief that illness had a physical and rational explanation. Hippocrates also held the belief that the body must be treated as a whole and not just a series of parts.[142]

So, when a cure for cancer, or any other disease is mentioned here, it's a re-instatement of what Hippocrates observed thousands of years ago; giving our body what it needs, so the body can naturally heal itself.

Speaking of cancer, Dr. Otto Warburg, who was awarded a Nobel Prize for his research on cancer in 1931; and nominated for another in 1944, said this:

"There is no disease whose prime cause is better known, so that today ignorance is no longer an excuse that one cannot do more about prevention of cancer. But how long prevention will be avoided depends on how long the prophets of agnosticism will succeed in inhibiting the application of scientific knowledge in the field of cancer. In the meantime, millions of men and women must die of cancer unnecessarily."[143]

—Dr. Otto Warburg

NOTE: In 1900, cancer struck only 3% of Americans, whereas today it strikes over 40% of Americans.

Does this statement create any curiosity? It should! Dr. Warburg won his Nobel Prize more than 75 years ago. Why is cancer continuing

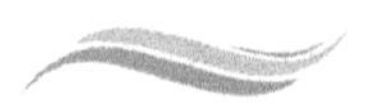

to skyrocket? Do we really know what causes cancer as Dr. Warburg suggests? If so, why is this not public knowledge? What ever happened to Dr. Warburg, why has nobody ever heard of him?

This is an exciting principle to talk about! ***What if***...these "theories" contain the cause, prevention, and ***cure for cancer***, which now kills over 40% of all Americans, also the prevention and cure for many other diseases, like heart disease which kills 50% of all Americans? ***What If***...in these theories we have found the key to the ***Secret to the Fountain of Youth?*** We all will die someday, but we can significantly slow down the aging process if we adhere to sound principles of healthy living.

These are called "theories" because they are not yet proven facts through science, but much of what we are now teaching in universities and practicing in medicine as "fact", is also theory.[144] Remember, when it is said and done, we really only understand a very small percentage (maybe 10%) of what actually happens in our bodies.[145]

"Only 15% of medical interventions are supported by solid scientific evidence…this is because only one percent of the articles in medical journals are scientifically sound, and partly because many treatments have never been assessed at all."

—Richard Smith – *British Medical Journal*[146]

There is a well-known "alternative" cancer treatment clinic in San Diego and Mexico named the Gerson Clinic. They use an approach that centers around fresh organic vegetables, fruits, whole grains, supplementation, and elimination of virtually all toxins. A study of the Gerson method evaluated the five-year survival rates of 153 melanoma patients. It found that 100 percent of the patients with Stage One, and Stage Two cancers receiving the Gerson therapy survived, but only 70 percent of the conventionally treated patients. For patients with cancer that had spread to other sites close to the original cancer (Stage

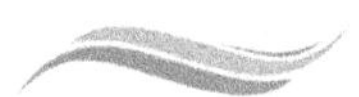

Three), 70 percent of the Gerson patients survived, verses 41 percent of those treated with allopathic medical techniques. Of those patients whose cancer had spread to distant parts of their body (Stage Four), 39 percent of the Gerson patients were still alive, compared to just 6 percent of those treated with conventional therapy. This result is truly amazing; there were six patients alive on the Gerson treatment for every one patient receiving conventional chemotherapy and radiation.[147]

So, let's talk about these theories and how they work. *Free radicals* are molecules that are missing an electron in their outer shell. Because these free radical molecules are missing an electron they are in an unstable state. They are positively charged, because electrons carry a negative charge, and if molecules are missing an electron, it creates a positively charged free radical. They go throughout our bodies causing problems. They attach onto healthy cell walls in our bodies and steal electrons from healthy molecules that are not missing electrons, ones that are in a stable state. After being attacked by the free radicals they become free radicals themselves because the free radical steals their electron, thus making the one being attacked now a molecule that is missing an electron, a free radical; thus, it is like a wild game of tag throughout our body. These free radicals attack our DNA, which are the building blocks of our bodies, the system by which you remain you as your body regenerates itself every few weeks.[148] What is the result? Nothing good. Where do these free radicals come from? Free radicals come from many sources, including by-products of metabolism, pollution, the sun, stress, and cigarette smoke.[149]

Well, what is cancer? In simple terms it is a good cell, gone bad, that replicates.[150] If free radicals can mess up healthy cell walls and can attack our DNA, the replicating system of our body, doesn't it make logical sense that they can cause cancer?[151]

Now, cancer is thought to be multi-causal, meaning there is likely more than one pathway that causes the disease.[152] But there is

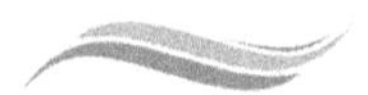

common agreement that this attack on healthy cells, and our DNA, is thought to be a primary pathway that leads to the disease.[153]

"Carcinogenesis, the process that leads to cancer, is believed to occur in a series of steps. It is a multistage process that begins with precancerous cellular damage that gradually proceeds to more malignant changes. The first step is the development of cellular abnormalities, which eventually leads to cancer."

—Dr. Joel Fuhrman, *Eat to Live*, p.77

Dr. Otto Warburg won his Nobel Prize for discovering that *cancer cells cannot grow in an oxygen rich environment.*[154] What causes an oxygen rich environment? How do we get more oxygen to our cells? When we exercise, we run more oxygen through our body. We can also do it through the food we eat; if we eat foods and drink water that are more alkaline, we bring more oxygen to our cells. A pH of 10.0 is 10 times more alkaline than a pH of 9.0, and 100 times more alkaline as a pH of 8.0..[155] There is a simple 5 cent test to determine where your urine is at on the pH scale. Just get a piece of litmus paper and test your urine. Our pH varies in different parts of our bodies, and at different times of the day depending on what we eat, if we exercise, or our stress levels. Some areas need to maintain a very strict pH for our survival, and other areas vary dramatically.[156] If one area is abnormally out of balance, it makes sense that it draws from other areas to regulate itself, and thus one area can affect other areas.

Albert Einstein and Dr. Otto Warburg were good friends, and Einstein greatly admired Warburg's research. Einstein even wrote Warburg a letter imploring him to not continue his service in the German Army in World War I because of his value to humanity.[157]

"Warburg was to medicine and biochemistry as Einstein was to physics. The only difference is that the prejudiced low lives in medicine are still obstructing the discoveries of Otto Warburg; namely, that cancer is a disease of respiratory impairment; namely, oxygen

deficiency to living cells, whereas the physics community has been intelligent enough to recognize what Einstein was saying, although they too, have sought to ignore the contributions of others to relativity, like those of Lorentz and Poincare, and exaggerate those of Einstein. Warburg, like Einstein, was a genius level scientist."

—Winfield J. Abbey[158]

Much of modern medicine dismisses Dr. Warburg's theories and his Nobel Prize and says he is a quack. They have taken cells and injected them with oxygen and do not get the same results as he did, so they say it is all quackery and doesn't work.[159] Has anyone ever thought that maybe our bodies just don't work this way? Maybe the only way to get more oxygen to our cells in a way that is usable is through exercise and an alkaline nutrition program?

Do free radicals and an acidic PH affect one another? Yes. Free radicals cause a more acidic environment in our body.[160] Stress also creates free radicals and an acidic PH in our body.[161] They are inseparably connected to one another. Future research will likely uncover a better understanding of all this, but right now it is obvious they do affect one another.

In the book, *The Calcium Factor*, by Robert Barefoot and Dr. Carl Reich, Robert talks about free radicals and the pH balance theory, and the importance of minerals to our bodies. Robert talks about the importance of minerals in maintaining an alkaline pH in our body; he mentions the Hopi Indians of Arizona and the Hunza of Northern Pakistan, and others, where cancer is almost non-existent.[162] He says the major difference in their lifestyle from others is the elevation these people live at which is usually 8,500 feet and above, thus avoiding the free radicals in pollution, and the abundance of minerals in the water supply and in their irrigation. Dr. Joel Wallach, a 1991 Nobel Prize nominee, also talks extensively about several groups of people who regularly have people living between 120-140 years of age that also exhibit many of the same lifestyle characteristics.[163]

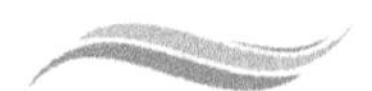

"By also using these minerals to raise the pH to above the 7.4 range to a pH of 8.5, the cancer cells would die while the healthy cells would thrive: thus, once again verifying the observations of both the turn-of-the-century doctors and men like Dr. Reich. Unfortunately, before the physician can practice preventive medicine, he must prove that nutritional therapy works to the satisfaction of the governing regulators who already have refused to examine the massive documentation available, most of which was provided by the world's best scientists, some of whom won Nobel Prizes for their efforts. In other words, the American Medical Association just refuses to listen to logic, preferring to tread the beaten path of escalating disease treated by unnatural and expensive man-made chemicals. The cost of this stance is massive human suffering, and premature death of millions of Americans."[164]

—*The Calcium Factor*

What if 90% of all our diseases or illnesses we face in our society are the result of *lifestyle* not genetics? The foods we eat, the thoughts we think, the presence or absence of exercise...our *behavior?* If we believed this, we might accept more responsibility for our personal health and treat our bodies with a lot more respect.

There is a great story out by Dr. Loraine Day.[165] She is a cancer survivor. Her cancer started with a breast tumor and spread to her lymphatic system and eventually all over her body. She is a medical doctor but refused normal chemotherapy and radiation treatment and was to the point of just a few days to live, with huge tumors all over her body. She used all natural methods to get rid of her cancer, and in her videos and tapes she outlines a 10-step program that she says is God's Health Plan that has been around for thousands of years, and is ***FREE***, compared to most of our modern medicine that has been around for about 50 years, and is *very* expensive. Dr. Day says these 10 Steps will give your body what it needs to beat cancer, and most other diseases, almost every time.[166] The term most is used because

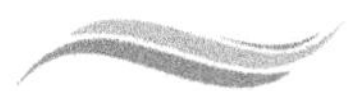

none of us is perfect, and we all fall short in some way, but God's Health Plan works 100% of the time. God wants us to be healthy and free of disease. We glorify Him when we are healthy. Would you like to know the 10 steps of God's Health Plan?

God's 10-Step Health Plan

1. Nutrition – centered around fruits, vegetables, and whole grains
2. Exercise – everyday
3. Water – 10 glasses a day
4. No Chemicals – environment & in food
5. Sunlight – everyday
6. Fresh Air – everyday
7. Proper Rest at the Proper Time
8. Trust in God – not in the wisdom of man which is foolishness with God
9. Have an Attitude of Gratitude – realize how blessed we really are
10. Benevolence – reach out and help others

Dr. Day has video tapes and CD's you can buy and listen to. They are great for anyone you know who has cancer, or any other chronic disease, or just wants to avoid these terrible diseases, which is hopefully everyone. You can get them on her website, DrDay.com. This is fascinating information from a very credible lady. She's been Chief of Staff in Orthopedics at San Francisco General Hospital and has trained thousands of physicians.

Have you ever thought much about *how* we get the diseases that actually kill most people here in America? Do we catch them, or do we develop them? We develop cancer and heart disease. They are

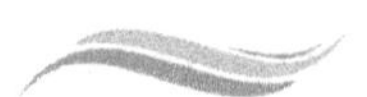

not a bacteria or virus that we catch; we do these things to ourselves. Yes, the enemy really is us. Some people are offended by these statements and say, how can you say a young child can cause their own cancer, or developed their own Type I diabetes? They are too young to cause anything, which is maybe true, but what about the lifestyle and the toxins they have been exposed to up to that point in their lives? What about their parents, and grandparent's lifestyle, and the toxins they were exposed to during the course of their lives, and when their mother was pregnant? Some say this is heredity, what we are exposed to through our progenitors, but most of us can stop this heredity through our lifestyle. Yes, some people are more susceptible to a certain disease than others, but we can *stop the cycle*.

Do you know how many free radicals are in one puff of a cigarette? About *100 trillion*. How can our bodies withstand that kind of free radical damage? They can't. Research is also linking free radical damage and an acidic pH to plaque build-up in our arteries, which causes heart disease. This kills 50% of all Americans. So, just with these 2 diseases, cancer & heart disease, almost all American deaths are linked to free radicals and an acidic pH. They are also linking free radical damage to premature aging. Why do people who smoke or sit out in the sun too much look 10 years older than others their same age? Sun is a good thing, it gives us the Vitamin D that we need, but be careful because the sun produces free radicals, just like smoking does. Smoking is so obviously bad for us it must be stopped. Do young people who smoke have any idea what they are doing to their marvelous bodies, and their entire being, BodyMindSpirit?

The American Cancer Society says about 70% of cancer is directly related to our *nutrition*.[167] Why is this not translated to us as Americans, or to our physicians? We hear about it in soft ways like the following quote, but we need to hear it above all the other noise out there in the marketplace because it is the answer to our problems.

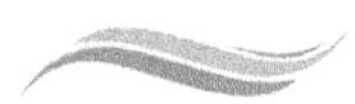

"Cancer is the second leading cause of illness and death in the United States. Good nutrition is important to preventing, dealing with, and surviving cancer. The cause of most cancers is still unclear, but a healthy lifestyle can improve your odds and help maintain your health during treatment. In particular, certain foods can assist in helping to protect you from colon cancer. Try adding these foods to your eating plan for better health – Whole-grain breads, pasta, cereal and brown rice, dried beans, fresh fruits and vegetables, and foods low in fat. High-fiber foods help move waste through your digestive tract faster, so harmful substances don't have much contact with the lining of the intestine. High-fiber foods are also rich in phytonutrients, which appear to protect against several forms of cancer."

—American Dietetic Association

Our body's natural protection against free radicals are nutrients called *antioxidants*; they are produced outside the body so they have to be taken in the form of food or supplements.[168] The more well-known antioxidants are: vitamins A, B-complex, C, D & E, selenium, zinc, glutathione, pycnogenol, carotenoids, and flavonoids.[169] These antioxidants have extra electrons to give up to neutralize the free radicals so they don't go around causing havoc in our bodies. They stop that wild game of tag and render the free radicals harmless...isn't our body amazing?

There are also many other anti-cancerous substances in natural plant food, and more are being discovered everyday...there are over *10,000 phytonutrients* (Phyto=plant) *in just one tomato.*[170] We simply do not understand all the benefits of whole natural food.

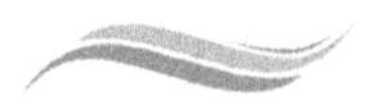

"The most compelling evidence of the last decade has indicated the importance of protective factors, largely unidentified, in fruits and vegetables."

—Walter C. Willett, M.D., Ph.D., chairman of the Department of Nutrition at Harvard's School of Public Health, and a speaker at the American Association for Cancer Research

Here's a small sample of some of the anti-cancerous substances found on fruits and vegetables: Allium compounds, Allyl sulfides, Anthocyanins, Caffeic acid, Catechins, Coumarins, Dithiolthiones, Ellagic acid, Ferulic acid, Flavonoids, Glucosinolatesm Indoles, Isoflavones, Isothiocyanates, Lignans, Liminoids, Pectins, Perillyl alcohol, Phenolic acids, Phytoesterols, Polyacetylenes, Polyphenols, Protease inhibitors, Saponins, Sulphorophane, Sterols, Terpenes.[171]

"The list above is only a small sample of beneficial compounds, and more are being discovered everyday...There are simply too many protective factors that work synergistically to expect significant benefit from taking a few isolated substances. These beneficial compounds have overlapping and complementary mechanisms of action. They inhibit cellular aging, induce detoxifying enzymes, bind carcinogens in the digestive tract, and fuel cellular repair mechanisms."

—Dr. Joel Fuhrman, *Eat to Live*

So, basically, we need to eat a variety of whole natural plant food to get all the phytonutrients that we need to inhibit or repair cellular damage and prevent cancer.[172] As with all diseases, it is much easier to prevent cancer than cure it.[173] Cellular wall and DNA damage occurs over a period of many years.[174] Take the proper precautions now to prevent this terrible disease *before* it happens to you or a loved one.

Take a guess, if you don't know already, what foods are most antioxidant rich, and the best foods to get our body to more of an alkaline state? ***Fruits, and vegetables.*** Alcohol, fat, sugar, meat

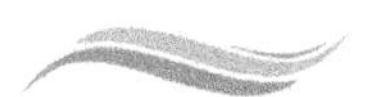

and dairy products are low in most antioxidants and will cause our body to become more acidic, thus one of the reasons why they should be eaten sparingly. The following is a short list of some of the acidic vs. alkaline foods:[175]

Foods that are Acidic	Foods that are Alkaline
Bacon	Almonds
White Bread	Avocados
Cheese	Green Beans
Ice Cream	Spinach
White Pasta	Apricots
Yoghurt	Oranges
Soft Drinks	Carrots
Beef	Watermelon
Coffee	Potatoes
Shrimp	Green Lettuce
Chicken	Tomatoes
Crackers	Cherries
Milk	Berries
Turkey	Grapes/Raisins
Butter	Squash
Processed Cereals	Broccoli
Pork	Cantaloupe
Alcohol	Pears

Your thoughts will also have a dramatic effect on your free radicals and bodies pH; stress, anger and other negative emotions will create many more free radicals and cause your bodies overall pH to lower. There are studies that say our *thoughts can have a more profound effect on our body's pH than our food.*[176] Exercise helps prevent or relieve negative emotions. Use the WAVE and other principles taught in this book. Test this out for yourself. Get a bunch of pH test strips and test yourself regularly. See if these principles are true. Read all you can so you become informed, so these principles become a part of your daily thoughts and life patterns.

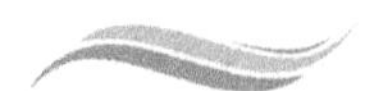

Anyone who has worked in the health and fitness industry frequently hears amazing stories about good nutrition and exercise, just like the Dr. Loraine Day story. One man said his wife was diagnosed with cancer with only a couple months to live. She had large open sores all over her body from the cancer. He had heard about some of these wellness resorts and some of the remarkable stories about patients there. So, he and his wife figured they had nothing to lose and would give it a shot. At the time of telling this story she was still alive, that was *14 years* after she was told she had 2 months to live. The wellness resort put her on a very strict nutrition program, high in fruits, vegetables, whole grains, and had her supplementing with vitamins and minerals, antioxidants.[177] Again, isn't our body amazing if we feed it the nutrition it needs?

"He who does not know food, how can he understand the diseases of man?"

—Hippocrates

Could the answer to most of our problems really be this simple?

What happens if we don't get the phytonutrients or antioxidants we need? Or are exposed to too many free radicals, and our bodies become acidic? We will be much more likely to get cancer, heart disease, look old, and have all the problems associated with free radicals and an acidic PH; we become an environment where illness and disease will thrive.[178] Like previously mentioned, the major food source of antioxidants is fruit and vegetables; antioxidants cause the marvelous colors in fruits and vegetables.[179] This is another reason why any diet that preaches against fruit and vegetables is on the wrong path. *Only 10%* of Americans daily nutrition is coming from fruits and vegetables, and some are telling us not to eat them?[180] Obviously they do not understand or believe in the Free Radical / PH Balance Theories. Why else would they tell us to not eat our fruits? Yes, some fruits and vegetables are higher on the glycemic index than

others, and some have more nutrition than others, but, if we focus your nutrition on all the glorious fruits and vegetables we can find, we will be fine, because they even each other out, and it's much more important to have them than not. Many people get so focused on the insignificant tangents, that they do not see the big picture and forget what's most important.

Some would ask that if free radicals are caused by our bodies' metabolism, and if exercise creates more free radicals, is exercise then really good for us? Exercise is discussed extensively in the 7 Principles of Exercise; we were created to be physically active, it's best for our overall health and well-being. It relieves stress and lowers our body's pH, so our bodies are less likely to break down and become diseased. It gets more oxygen to our cells and will likely help prevent cancer cells from growing.[181] Also, because of the marvelous way God set things up, we can get all the antioxidants we need through our nutrition to combat the free radical damage we experience from exercise. But we should be aware that our bodies are experiencing more free radicals from exercise, and take extra steps to insure we are getting all the antioxidants we need.[182] We need both, exercise and good nutrition.

Dr. Andrew Weil, founder and Director of the Arizona Center of Integrative Medicine, and Dr. Dean Ornish, the founder and President of the non-profit Preventive Medicine Research Institute, and a clinical professor at the University of California, San Francisco, have *thousands* of other physicians across the country following their preventive approaches to health care.[183] They have created this following because their methods make sense, and they work. They talk about how with the health care system in America doctors are incentivized to spend little time with patient's and recommend prescription drugs and surgeries, because those are what they get reimbursed for.

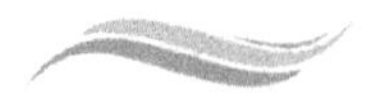

If you think about it, there are only two ways to solve our health care crisis:

1. Spend less money
2. Make people healthier

Which one makes the most sense? Obviously, it would be great to lower our costs, and we should do everything we can to be as efficient and fair as possible. But the reality is it takes huge amounts of money to run our hospitals, and doctors go to college for almost a decade and will likely never be paid nominal salaries. So, the likely choice is *let's help people be healthier!* ***What if*** we could drop health care costs in *half* in 5 short years by bringing prevention to the forefront of American's minds?[184] Would this help our economy? Would it create more jobs? Would people live healthier, happier lives? Yes, yes, YES!

Another thing to mention when we talk about free radicals is trying to limit the amounts of toxic chemicals that we are exposed to. If you take a more in-depth look at those cultures which regularly have people live to 120-140 years, there are a couple distinguishing characteristics.[185] First, they generally live in elevations above 8,000 feet, and second, they drink and irrigate their soils with water from the mountains that has a lot of minerals in it. We will talk more about minerals when we talk about supplementation, but what about the elevation? Logic tells us that they are exposed to far less chemicals and pollutants than we are. What exact cultures are we talking about?

In a January 1973 edition of National Geographic entitled, "Search for The Oldest People", provided examples of many of these cultures, including the Abkhazians from Georgia (high in the mountains), the Hunzas of Pakistan (high in the mountains), and the Vilcabambas of Ecuador (high in the mountains). This list was quickly expanded to include the Bamas in China (high in the mountains), the Azerbaijan's (high in the mountains), the Tibetans (high in the mountains), and the Titicaca of Peru (high in the mountains) ...With all the above

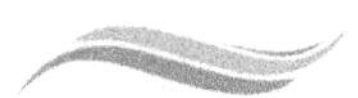

cultures, disease does not exist: [virtually] no cancer, no heart disease, no diabetes, no Alzheimer's, no arthritis, etc. These cultures have no mental health disorders and no doctors. They also live decades longer than we do in North America, and their aging process is dramatically slower."[186]

When these people move to places like North America, their rates of disease climb to exactly equal our rates.[187] It is clearly lifestyle, not genes, that cause disease. Particularly important are the presence of whole foods full of minerals and other phytonutrients, the absence of toxins, and exercise. Let's learn the lessons of history and learn from the world's oldest living people!

What else can we do to protect ourselves? Our skin is the largest organ in our body. Doesn't it make sense that we should be very careful not only about what we put on the inside of our body, but also the outside? Our skin breathes. It moves nutrients and toxins in and out of the body. If you don't believe this, try rubbing a strong oil like eucalyptus on the bottom of your feet. Almost immediately you will be able to taste the oil in your mouth. What does this tell us? Not only do we need to be very cautious about what we eat and drink, but also what we expose our bodies to through our skin. It might be a good practice to not put anything on our skin that cannot be eaten or ingested.

The water you drink and shower with might be a good place to start. What is the quality of the water where you live? If it's really bad get some type of filtering device, not only for your drinking water, but also for your shower and bath water. There are water filtering devices in the marketplace that are great. Many are made by Japanese companies; you just hook the unit up to your kitchen sink. They also have a unit that is made for the whole house. About 1/3 of the homes in Japan have a unit like this. Basically, what it does is filter out the bad things in the water, like: fluoride, chlorine, and heavy metals like aluminum, and lead. Then it separates all the alkaline and acidic minerals in the water and allows you to choose how alkaline or acidic

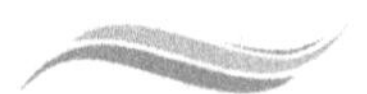

you want your water by simply touching a button. It is amazing. If your body is too acidic simply drink more alkaline water. You will feel when it is about the right pH for you.

Dr. Lorraine Day, Denise Austin, and many other health professionals say we should drink *10 glasses of water every day.*[188] But unfortunately most of the bottled water in the stores, and out of our faucets, is very acidic. Get a pH test kit and do a simple test for the water you drink to see how acidic or alkaline it is. Then you will have a better idea of what you are taking into your body. Do you think this unit would be in one out of every three homes if the Japanese people did not believe in the pH Theory, or if there was not significant scientific evidence that this device really works and helps to make people healthier? Most Americans haven't even heard of the pH Balance Theory, let alone have one of these units in their home. Why is that? Hopefully by the end of this book you will understand that most of the problems we have with our health care system is our own fault, we are way too focused on the wrong things. We can blame others, but the market is just giving us what we want and will buy. You can visit our website, Wave4Life.com for more information.

Be careful about carrying a cell phone in your pocket, or talking a lot on it unless you have an earpiece.[189] Also be cautious you about using a microwave oven, especially when cooking in plastics; take a little more time and heat things up on the stove.[190] Your toothpaste, shampoo, and make-up are also important.[191] Currently WAVE offers some personal care products that do not have the harsh chemicals, so you will have less exposure to toxins through these products. The product line will be expanded, you can log on to wave4life.com to see what is currently available.

Heavy metals can be a big problem, especially if people are dealing with arthritis or other auto-immune diseases.[192] There is a great book entitled, *Overcoming Arthritis*, by Dr. David Brownstein. This is a must read for anyone who suffers from arthritis, or any other

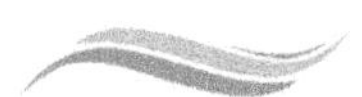

autoimmune disease. Good nutrition is most important for most people, but if some have been exposed to large amounts of toxic heavy metals, they may be causing the problems. Heavy metals include: • Mercury • Arsenic • Cadmium • Lead • Nickel • Aluminum

Heavy metals are toxins that can come from a variety of sources, including industrial pollutants in the air, water and soil, our food supply, and dental fillings.[193] There isn't time here to talk about all of these, but it's important to at least mention mercury.

"The U.S. Department of Health and Human Services lists mercury as the third most hazardous substance known to mankind. The World Health Organization states that there is no minimum level of mercury that does not cause harm. The number one source of mercury poisoning is dental fillings. Dental amalgams (fillings) contain approximately 50% mercury as well as other metals, including nickel. The World Health Organization estimates that the largest source of mercury in humans comes from fillings implanted by dentists. The amount of mercury from fillings is over 10 times more than all the other sources combined. Mercury is easily absorbed from the fillings in the mouth. It can be released as a vapor in the mouth, and chewing exacerbates its release...I cannot fathom why dentists still use mercury fillings when the danger and toxicity of mercury is a well-known fact. It is my opinion that mercury amalgams should be banned, as has been done in some European countries."[194]

— Dr. David Brownstein

Mercury has also been used for years as a preservative in vaccines.[195] Dr. Brownstein says a recent study says that each year 60,000 children in the U.S. are born with neurological problems resulting from exposure to mercury, and that newborns can acquire mercury toxicity from their mothers.[196] He suggests that those who suffer from arthritis and other autoimmune diseases may want to replace their dental fillings.[197] But the removal of mercury fillings is an expensive process and one that must be done with great care. A

dentist who is knowledgeable about the dangers of mercury can be found by contacting the following organizations:

1. DAMS Organization: (800) 311-6265
2. International Academy of Oral Medical Toxicology (IAOMT): (407) 299-4149

It is also wise to have a really good air filtering system in our homes, or maybe just in the rooms your family sleeps in if you cannot afford it throughout the entire house. There are lots of toxins in our air supply, from car pollution, and industrial plants. You might not be able to do anything about your work environment, but something can be done about our homes, where we sleep and spend much of our time each day. WAVE will offer home air filtering systems on our website or recommend someone in your local area that offers a good quality product.

Some say it is better to *not* put sunscreens on our skin because of all the toxic chemicals that most have in them which are harmful.[198] Is it better to deal with more free radical damage than expose ourselves to the toxins in the sunscreen? You will have to read, become informed, and be the judge of the importance of all these things in your life. It does makes sense that we should be cautious about the toxins we expose ourselves to, especially since those cultures in which people regularly live to 120 -140 years, where cancer and heart disease are less than 1%, are those who live in almost toxic-free environments. One thing is a given, free radicals are real, and an acidic pH causes problems. Just be aware of all this as you go about your daily activities.

QUESTION EVERYTHING?
MOM, DO FRUITS AND VEGETABLES PREVENT SKIN CANCER?
QETommy.com

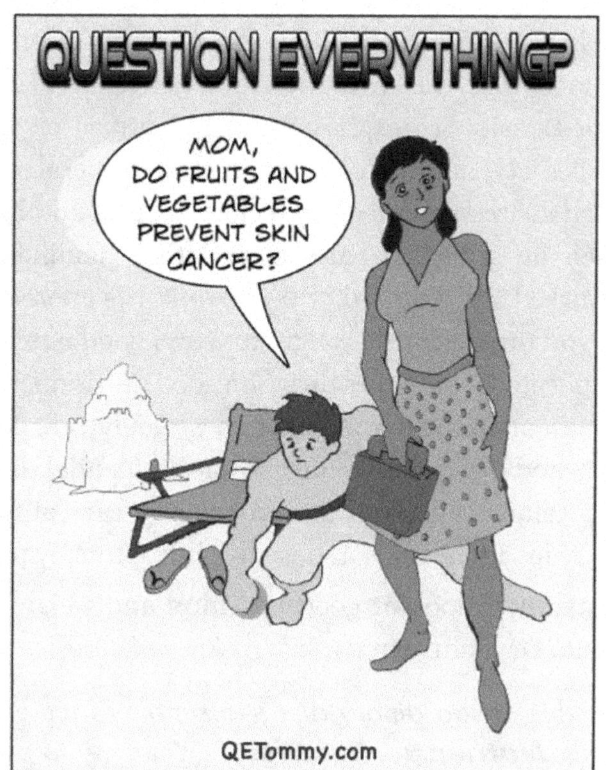

PRINCIPLE #4
EAT HIGH DENSITY FOODS

Is feeling satisfied, no obesity and no disease really possible?

In the marvelous book, *Eat to Live*, by Dr. Joel Fuhrman, he uses a common-sense approach to nutrition that is backed up by undeniable research and science. Dr. Fuhrman is a licensed physician and has treated thousands of his patients and achieved absolutely amazing results. Many of his patients are losing 20 pounds of body fat the first month on his program and never gain it back.[199]

The basis of Dr. Fuhrman's approach is a Nutrient Density Chart, in which he lists the foods that have the most nutrition per calorie, down to the foods with the lowest nutrition per calorie. He rates foods with Nutrient Density Scores, based upon identified phytochemicals, antioxidant activity, and total vitamin and mineral content. Dr. Fuhrman then shares great tasting recipes that he and his wife have created which he gives his patients and their families.[200] He has personally worked with over *10,000 patients*. His approach is one of logic. When you think about it weight loss and good nutrition are just not that complicated; our bodies thrive on good nutrition. If we eat food that is high in calories and low in nutrition we get fat, are hungry all the time, get sick, and live far below our physical potential. If we eat food that is low in calories and high in nutrition, we can eat to our hearts content, stay thin, are healthy, and we live life optimally physically.

The best way to look at good nutrition and weight loss is this simple formula Dr. Fuhrman uses:

"The key to this extraordinary diet is a simple formula: ***H = N/C (Health = Nutrients/ Calories)*** *...Your key to permanent weight loss is to eat predominantly those foods that have a high proportion of nutrients to calories."*[201]

—Eat to Live

This is great because it is so simple, easy to understand, and it makes perfect sense. If we don't get what we need our bodies break down or we die early deaths. This is what we are as a nation right now, over fed and under nourished. We eat foods that have little or no nutritional value, and then we wonder why we have so many problems. We can blame things on our genetics, but a much more logical explanation is our poor nutrition. We are simply not getting what we need to sustain life and function optimally.

Let's take a look at Dr. Fuhrman's marvelous Nutrient Density Chart:[202]

Order of Nutrient Density in Foods –
(highest nutrient density = 100 points,
lowest nutrient density = 0 points)

100 points = Raw leafy green vegetables (darker green has more nutrients)
97 points = Solid green vegetables (raw, steamed, or frozen)
50 points = non-green, non-starchy vegetables
48 points = Beans, legumes (cooked, canned, or sprouted)
45 points = Fresh fruits
35 points = Starchy vegetables
22 points = Whole grains
20 points = Nuts and seeds

---

15 points = Fish
13 points = Fat-free dairy
11 points = Wild meats and fowl
11 points = Eggs
8 points = Red meat
4 points = Full-fat dairy
3 points = Cheese
2 points = Refined grains (white flour)
1 point = Refined oils
0 points = Refined sweets

Where is most of your nutrition coming from, above the line, or below the line? If you said above the line, you are to be congratulated. If you said below you need to make some changes.

"Appetite is not controlled by the weight of the food but by fiber, nutrient density, and caloric density...it's pretty clear which foods will let you feel full with the least number of calories – fruits and green vegetables. Green vegetables, fresh fruits, and legumes will take the gold, silver, and bronze medals. Nothing else in the field is even close.[203]"

—Dr. Joel Fuhrman, *7X NY Times Best Selling Author*

The other thing that makes sense about this nutrient density approach is it makes it easy to empower people, to educate but not dictate. Thus, teaching people correct principles and letting them figure out for themselves what foods they will eat, which is the best way to help people.[204] To read more visit drfuhrman.com.

This principle might lead to a discussion about supplementation, and how we can just add nutrients back into our foods to make them more nutritious. You can get lots of specific nutrients and no calories with supplementation. The basic problem with this is we are only just beginning to understand all the nutrition that is in whole unprocessed food, directly from Mother Earth. As mentioned earlier, scientists have discovered over 10,000 phytonutrients in a single tomato, and this may be just the beginning.[205] It is impossible to replicate whole food in the laboratory. Mother Nature has given us the amazing qualities of whole food with thousands of nutrients packed in perfect proportions, working in beautiful harmony, and true synergy. Supplementation will never take the place of good nutrition; only maybe add something to it.

The question then is, can we get everything we need from our food supplies? The answer is likely yes, but we will need to eat mostly organic food or grow our own, eat a wide variety of fruits, vegetables, whole grains, legumes, nuts, and seeds.... this is exactly what is recommended in this book. You also might need to juice with fruits and vegetables. The next question then becomes, do most people have the desire or training to be this dedicated in their nutrition? Or more importantly, can they work into it? The answer again is yes. WAVE's desire as a company is to help Americans find the truth and work into it.

Having said all this let's talk a bit about supplementation. There is the chance that even if you are one of those who lives this lifestyle completely, you still might be lacking in some of the 90 nutrients we need every day.[206] Why? Because our soils and foods are becoming

increasingly depleted of nutrients, and we are exposed to more toxic chemicals each year.[207] This is why it is recommended that people supplement.

Many times, our soils are not allowed to rest as Mother Nature intended. We think we can just put our man-made chemicals into the soils and they will be OK, but some of our farmlands are so depleted that weeds will not even grow in them. If we plant in them for 7 years, a good practice is to let them rest for 7 years, to let them fill back up with nutrients.[208] We must rest our soils to let the nutrients from rains and natural fertilizers settle back into the soils. This is one of the distinguishing characteristics of those cultures whose citizens live so long. Their soils are irrigated naturally with the glacial milk, which is runoff from the mountains full of minerals.[209] Most of our food soils are fertilized with cheap man-made fertilizers, which many times make the crops look big and pretty, so they are aesthetically appealing, and people buy them, but they are desperately lacking in nutrition.[210]

The result for us is lack of nutrition and poor health, even if our eating habits are really good. This is very sad situation. Buy organic. Not to say that organic food is always better than the regular grocery store varieties, but it definitely has less of the toxic chemicals and is generally more nutritious.[211] But do some reading on your own. Become proficient at reading labels and asking questions. Or better yet, don't buy anything with a label on it! Become nutritionally educated.

It used to be that we could get all the nutrition we needed from eating healthy food bought at the regular grocery stores. Times have changed. Even 10 years ago scientists were telling us all we need to do is eat healthy, that we don't need supplements, that they only create expensive urine.[212] But most have since changed their opinions. There is just too much evidence that says otherwise.

What about pollution, toxic chemicals, and harsh pesticides? We are being bombarded with free radicals, and things that cause our

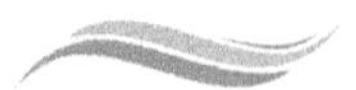

bodies to become acidic on a daily basis. Eat as much raw organic food as possible, center your nutrition around whole grains, fruits and vegetables, which includes legumes, nuts and seeds, and supplement.

With all the myriad of supplements out there in the marketplace, how do you know what to get? This is where WAVE can help.

Before deciding to represent any nutritional supplement WAVE did a lot of research and has decided to go with the supplement line called, LifeZone.[213] They are formulated by Dr. Janeel Henderson, who is a biochemist, and the daughter of world-famous Albion Lab founder, Dr. Harvey Ashmead. Dr. Ashmead became world famous during World War II for making Penicillin bio-available.[214] He is the one who made it usable to the human body. After the War he then spent the rest of his life (he died in 1998) on mineral research. Why? ***Minerals*** are a key ingredient to most reactions in our bodies, and many times the limiting factor to whether certain processes actually happen.[215] Dr. Ashmead formed Albion Laboratories in 1956, which is known world-wide as the foremost authority in mineral nutrition.[216] They have over 100 International patents on the chelation process of their minerals.[217] Dr. DeWayne Ashmead, Harvey's son, has been on C-SPAN with former President George Bush Jr., and former President Jimmy Carter, where he was invited to speak on the depletion of nutrients in our soils, fortification in our foods, and their patented chelated minerals.[218]

Basically, what Albion has done with minerals is replicate the processes of our body in the lab.[219] It's a bit technical, but it is important for you to understand it. When our body ingests a mineral, the molecular structure is so large that is has to be changed to a smaller form in to be absorbed, and become bioavailable, which means it is used at the cellular level. The mineral actually bonds to an amino acid, the basic elements of a protein, and the molecule becomes small enough to become bioavailable for your body to be able to use it as nutrition. There is an important difference between minerals being absorbed and bioavailable. When you buy supplements be cautious.

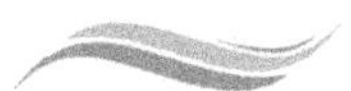

Some supplements can be very toxic to your body when taken in certain levels. Supplements that are absorbed but not bioavailable can cause problems. They can be deposited in your joints, muscles, and can go throughout your system causing problems.[220]

This is why bioavailability is so important, especially with minerals. Iron deficiency anemia is a huge health problem among menstruating women.[221] The doctors are in a "Catch 22." Do they give them more iron supplements in which the absorption is very low, maybe 5-10%, and have all the rest (90%) floating around in their body causing problems? Iron is very toxic at certain levels. So, what's the answer?

The Albion Chelates can certainly help. This is why Dr. Harvey Ashmead spent his life on mineral nutrition research. Minerals are critical to the health of every human on the earth. Albion has taken the process your body uses and replicates it outside the body in the lab. They completely wrap the mineral with an amino acid. A molecule is formed which is small enough to become used by our body, so our body absorbs it then uses it. It becomes bioavailable. This eliminates most of the problems associated with high doses of minerals, and minerals that are absorbed but not bioavailable.[222]

There are many companies that make many claims about their products. It is very hard to discern the truth of what they say about their products. There's a lot of research about many products, but never the amounts of research that there is about the Albion products, on a national and worldwide scale. There have been over 4,000 independent research studies on the Albion chelates that say they are the best in the world.[223] Most vitamins and mineral companies do their own research, and sometimes you really have to question the results because everyone seems to say they are the best. But with the Albion minerals these are *independent* studies, which means they are not getting money from the company, or are not associated with the company, so the likelihood of the results being biased, misrepresented, or untrue are much less; places like Harvard, Cornell, and U.C. Berkeley, have done the studies. The 100 U.S. patents should say something too. Also, the appointment of Dr. DeWayne Ashmead by former President George Bush, Jr. and former President Jimmy Carter on C-SPAN should add some validity to what they are doing.

Here's more information about the LifeZone products. There have only been eight product lines in Albion's 58-year history to receive the coveted Gold Medallion Award. LifeZone has received this award.[224] The LifeZone products are safe and have been on the market for many years.[225] They do not believe in mega-doses of nutrients. If the bioavailability is there you don't need those huge doses.

You can read more about these nutrients and specifically what they do online, but be assured you will get the very best supplements available to protect your body from disease, premature aging, depletion of nutrients in our soils and foods, and modern-day pollution.

After saying all this about supplements please remember that *all* supplements are secondary to good nutrition and exercise. It's always amazing how many companies, organizations, and people get so excited about supplements, but give little or no attention to nutrition and exercise. Yes, supplements are important, but people take something like one amino acid, which is one of the 20 essential amino acids that our body needs for a complete protein, or they take a fruit juice, that has great antioxidant properties, and that's all they talk about or promote. Let's get a little perspective here. It might be the most essential or the limiting amino acid out of all 20, or the best fruit juice in all the world, but can you live just on that one nutrient, or that one juice, or just that supplement? No possible way.

It is understood that companies and people need to make a living, and most often their focus is not balance and achievement, BodyMindSpirit, like this book and WAVE's mission. But this is one of the reasons why we are having so many problems in our free

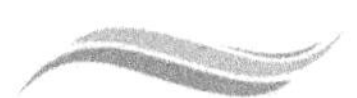

society. America and the freedoms and opportunities that this great nation brings to all of us are wonderful; it is the best nation in the world! WAVE might not have been able to get its start in any other nation in our modern world. This is one of the reasons why WAVE is stepping up to the plate to be known, out of love and gratitude for how very blessed we are to be here in America, and because people need a voice they can trust. People want to hear the truth, and they will get it. Not just in the physical aspect of our lives, but also in the mental and spiritual.

So, let's set the record straight; good nutrition is most important to good physical health. You can live on food alone with no exercise and no supplements. Exercise is maybe second most important as far as our health is concerned. Poor physical health might also be caused by a mental or spiritual ailment. Supplements are likely somewhere down the list. Always keep in mind that we need to consider our whole selves, in balance and synergy.

This is one of the reasons why our healthcare system is in such a sad state of affairs here in America. We take something that is a good thing, and through a lot of money, great marketing, and hype we make it up to be something it will never be, and we lose our perspective of what's most important. ***What If***...our focus in healthcare was on prevention, teaching people sound principles of nutrition and exercise, and treating our whole selves, BodyMindSpirit? We would likely be a much healthier and happier nation. Hopefully this book and WAVE will help you in some way to get back to the important basics of healthy living, help you get some of that perspective back.

Many of the modern-day athletes and bodybuilders claim to gain 20-30 pounds of solid muscle in a couple months because they have been working out; they have been working out and taking drugs! Our bodies do not respond that quickly. For a person in their mid 20's or 30's adding 10 pounds of muscle in a year is quite an accomplishment, especially if that person is active and in good shape.

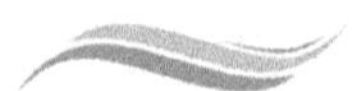

Yes, some people gain more muscle than others because of genetics. Maybe a teenager or someone who is still growing, has never lifted weights before, or has been away a long time might respond very quickly, but most all the others are taking drugs to grow that fast.

Recent reports say that over one million high school kids are currently using steroids. A 2006 NCAA survey of 20,000 college athletes found that more than half of college steroid users began using in high school. Fourteen percent began using even earlier.[226] This is so sad. Some mothers give their teenage daughters steroids in gymnastics and other sports to become more powerful. These drugs will cause addictions, health problems, and permanently change their bodies. Professional athletes who take these drugs to excel are called *cheaters*. People sell their souls to get ahead in life, and if everything is measured only by our temporal existence it might not seem so wrong, but there is so much more. The ban on steroids in professional baseball will likely not do too much good. Once the hype calms down many players just switch to things like Human Growth Hormone (HGH) that people can get from their doctors, and other drugs that do the same things as steroids.[227] Other athletes go on cycles of drugs during the off season when there is no testing. The governing bodies are not as unaware as they pretend to be; we need to be educated so we can do something about it. Why worry about what the athletes are doing? Because these are the people our kids idolize...maybe we should change this?

There are legal supplements out in the marketplace that will make dramatic improvements in a very short period of time, but most are not good for our bodies. Many people lose weight quickly by taking supplements that use caffeine and have other heart racing stimulants in them. They are not good for your body, stay away from them. If you have never taken these things before your body will literally shake. Can this be good for you?

Many women don't want to lift weights because they don't want to get big and look like the female bodybuilders. Women do not have the testosterone levels in their bodies to be able to look like this unless they are taking drugs. Yes, some women can build muscle very quickly, but that is maybe 1%, the rest could workout 8 hours a day and never build enough muscle to look like the female bodybuilders.

Are all people that have huge muscles like body builders on drugs? No, not all, but you lift weights and figure it out. If you are one of those rare women who do get big easily lifting weights, and you don't like the more athletic-type build, do less volume in your workout with more rest between sets. This will make you strong and make your muscles hard but will not add much size. Then drop your body fat down and you will become thinner. But be yourself, be proud of your genetics, it is a blessing to be able to build muscle quickly. It helps keep your body fat low and it's great for sport or just everyday life to be strong.

NOTE: Those persons with special needs, ones like pregnant and lactating women, should consult their physician before starting a supplement program. Also be cautious with children. Accidental overdose of iron-containing products is a leading cause of fatal poisoning in children less than six years of age. Please pay close attention to the labels of all products and follow their instructions before using them. Some people think because some is good more is better. This is not always the case; some vitamins and minerals are toxic in large doses. ***So, please use caution. Neither wave international, wave fitness, or any of its divisions, affiliates, officers, independent contractors, or employees will be held responsible in any way for any injuries or deaths due to the consumption or use of any nutritional supplements or products recommended above, or on the websites, so use caution.***

QUESTION EVERYTHING?
MOM, DO FISH IN THE OCEAN HAVE MERCURY IN THEM?
QETommy.com

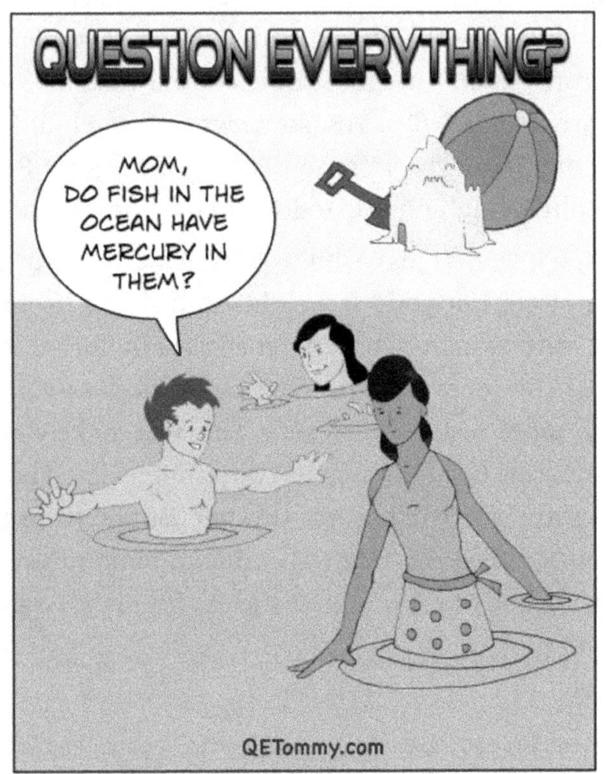

PRINCIPLE #5 – Words Of Wisdom

There are many

Utah is consistently one of the healthiest states in the nation, and the average active male member of the Church of Jesus Christ of Latter-day Saints, who occupy much of Utah, lives 14 years longer than the average male American. The women live 6 years longer than the average female American.[228] This is significant! These numbers cannot be ignored. What is causing this extended life? Members of the Church live by a code of health known as, The Word of Wisdom. Here are the Do's and Don'ts of The Word of Wisdom:

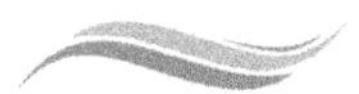

DO's

1. Eat every herb (vegetable) in its season
2. Eat every fruit in its season
3. All grain is ordained for the use of man (and woman)
4. Wheat is the staff of life
5. Eat meat sparingly and with thanksgiving

DON'TS

1. Smoke
2. Drink alcohol
3. Hot Drinks (coffee, tea)
4. Drugs (Illegal/ harmful)

Members have become famous for the don'ts, but even inside the faith few people follow the do's. Every fruit and vegetable in its season, all grain is ordained for the use of man, wheat is the staff of life, eat meat sparingly...does this go along with the low carb diets? No, in fact it's probably at the opposite end of the spectrum. No smoking, drugs or alcohol. Very simple, very straightforward, it works.

Most people agree that the healthiest things to eat, and what our nutrition should be centered around is; ***fruits, vegetables, and whole grains***, including legumes, nuts, and seeds. Everything else should be used sparingly. This makes it all easy, simple, and avoids all the confusion. We all have a tendency to make things way too complicated.

"Whole grains are very beneficial to your diet. They can help reduce your risk of heart disease, stroke, type 2 diabetes, several forms of cancer, and some gastrointestinal problems. Whole grain varieties include wheat, oats, corn and rye along with lesser-known ones like barley, spelt, grouts, wheat berries, millet, and flaxseed. Whole grains are found in cereals, crackers, and some whole grains can

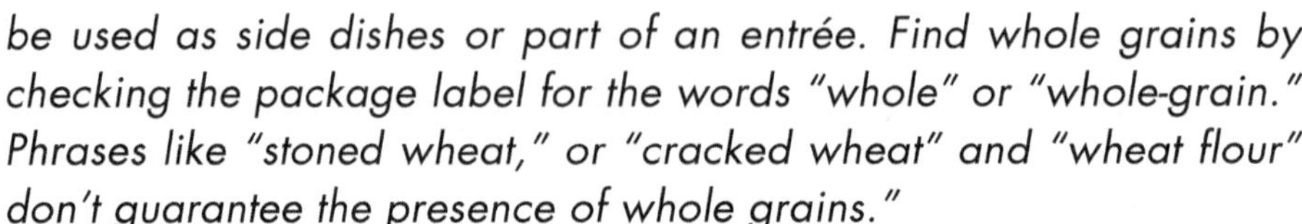

be used as side dishes or part of an entrée. Find whole grains by checking the package label for the words "whole" or "whole-grain." Phrases like "stoned wheat," or "cracked wheat" and "wheat flour" don't guarantee the presence of whole grains."

—American Dietetic Association

What other words of wisdom, groups of people, or cultures can we learn from? The 7th Day Adventists actually live longer than the Members of the LDS faith, and rank as some of the longest living people in the United States.[229] Their code of health is very similar, fruits, vegetables, and whole grains, except many don't eat any meat at all; they are vegetarians. These people are at the opposite ends of the spectrum of the low-carb diets. Maybe we should get the hint and forget about the low-carb craze, if we want to live a long and healthy life?

There are five-known cultures or groups of people in the world who regularly have people live between 120 and 140 years of age.[230] Dr. Joel Wallach, a 1991 Nobel Prize Nominee, has significant evidence of the people in these cultures living this long.[231] This is truly amazing, and what is even more interesting is they don't have most of the affluent diseases (cancer, heart disease) that kill almost 100% of all Americans.

Dr. Wallach says our genetic potential as humans is to live between 120 and 140 years. In his book, *Forbidden Cures*, he notes the common denominators of these people; the things he believes allow these people to live this long.[232]

1. The communities are found at elevations ranging from 8,500 feet to 14,000 feet in sheltered valleys. There is no heavy industry to pollute air, water, or food.
2. These people walk the hills, they exercise. ("The WAVE")
3. Their water source for drinking and irrigation comes from glacial melt and is known universally as "glacial milk" because

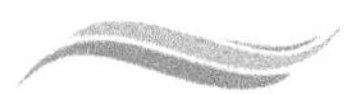

the highly mineralized water is opaque and whitish in color like milk.

4. Only natural fertilizers such as manure, plant debris, and glacial milk is employed.
5. Western allopathic medicine is not historically available to these cultures.

Dr. Wallach believes the *main* characteristic these people have that other cultures don't is they drink and irrigate their fields with glacial milk, run-off from the mountains, which is loaded with minerals. He says humans need *90 essential nutrients every day*, 60 minerals, 16 vitamins, 12 essential amino acids, and 3 fatty acids, and when we do not get them on a daily basis our bodies break down, we are inflicted with disease and die early deaths.[233] He also notes that these cultures center their nutrition around is fruits, vegetables, and whole grains. Some of these cultures do eat meat, but they are clean meats; no steroids, HGH, or other man-made chemicals added. Most of the animals feed off the land, or are grain fed, and there is no pollution in their food supply.

Another interesting book to read is *Mega Health*, written by Dr. Marc Sorenson, founder of The National Institute of Fitness. This is a resort where people can go to get healthy. The Fitness Institute puts their patients on nutrition that is very high in fruits, vegetables, and whole grains, supplements of minerals and antioxidants, a vigorous exercise program, and no meat or dairy (vegan). Dr. Sorenson's book, *Mega Health*, is one of the most highly researched books available. If you want to read about some amazing stories, read this book.

In Dr. Sorenson's book he says many people in healthcare give him the argument that disease is hereditary. He says he doesn't buy it. He says the same thing this book does. He notes cultures in the world today that have *less than 1% heart disease and cancer*, the two diseases that kill almost all Americans.[234] When these people move to

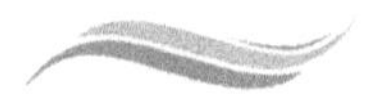

America, or other similar cultures, and eat like we do, their rates of these diseases increase to equal our numbers.

Let's talk a little more about our children. We are the examples in their life. If we don't get our own lives together, we are not giving our children much of a chance. Do you want your children growing up just like you? If you said yes, you are to be congratulated, especially if you are a healthy, happy person. Of course, we want our children to be a little better than we are, but we cannot expect this from them.

Our example is also where our children learn their lifestyle habits. From a health educator's perspective of 30+ years of experience, the toughest thing people ever do is change bad habits that they've established over a lifetime. This book is written to adults, but the primary target is our beloved children: these are those who will inherit the earth, and so much of what they will have and do will be because of us.

If you haven't seen the movie, *Super-Size Me*, rent it.[235] It is a documentary about a guy who goes on a 30-day diet of only McDonalds. He eats three meals a day there and eats everything on the menu at least once during the thirty days. According to the rules he has set, if the person taking the order asks him if he wants it "super-sized" he must say yes. In *thirty days,* his weight goes from 185 to about 220 lbs., his body fat goes from 11% to 18%, his heart healthy factors go from normal to out of control...basically his doctors tell him he is seriously risking his health if he continues to eat this way, even in this short 30-day period. The purpose here is not here to bash McDonald's; what Ray Krock and McDonald's has done is amazing. McDonald's is likely not any worse than any other fast-food restaurant, and you can eat somewhat healthy there just like you can at most other fast-food restaurants, but be careful. If you cannot make wise choices do not eat at these fast-food restaurants often, because if you eat poorly all the time you are going to have some serious health problems.

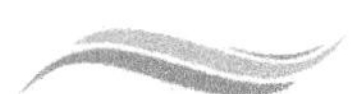

The most interesting part of the movie is about the children. They show what most kids eat for their school lunches – mostly junk food. They show a school that has adopted a really healthy lunch program. Their behavior problems have lowered, and their students' test scores and academic achievements have been raised. They also talk about how many schools are eliminating most of their physical education and nutrition education classes...not the right direction! With child obesity more than doubling since the late 70's, why would any educator in their right mind do away with physical education or nutrition classes? Parents need to demand these classes in schools and insist on healthy school lunches. The cost is not much different. This is not a financial issue; it is a health issue of what we want as parents. The junk food vending machines are a great revenue maker for many schools, but kids will buy the healthy stuff likely as much if it is available, especially if we educate them on why it is so important. We need to make choices as parents and educators that have the best interests of our kids in mind.

The system should not be so strict that it will not let someone have a birthday cake at school that has sugar in it. If we are consistently good, we can splurge and it's no big deal. But let's get rid of the soda pop and candy at school. Let's fill the machines with healthy snacks like raisins, trail mix, bottled water, 100% juice, whole-grain bars, celery, carrots, healthy sandwiches with whole-wheat bread, apples, oranges, etc.

Let's make lunches like those in the school that incorporated healthy lunches in *Super-Size Me*. They were awesome, and the kids loved them. Healthy food doesn't need to sacrifice in taste. Should the kids get a treat like a cookie or a small piece of cake at each meal? Yes, but let's make them as healthy as possible.

Every single kid at school needs at least an hour of physical activity every single day. If any parents want to fight about all this, let's bring out every study and all the statistics we can find to help

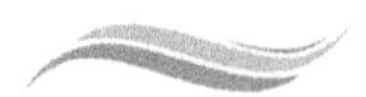

them to understand the importance of healthy nutrition and exercise. Let's hold nutrition and exercise education classes for parents. Schools that do this will see their school test scores rise not fall with this time away from their required curriculum, because their bodies and minds will function better when healthy.

If we are going to overcome our child obesity problems, we must *do something* about it. If we continue down the path we are on, things are going to only get worse. The cost of our healthcare can bankrupt our country and leave our children with many more problems than just obesity and a low quality and quantity of life.

The movie *Super-Size Me* then shows all the money that is spent on teaching our children about fast food, candy, pop, vs. the money that is spent on educating children about healthy eating. No thought of prevention – again.

The saddest part of the movie is when they hold up flash cards of famous people for a few children and ask them who they are. They have George Washington, who some get mixed up with Abraham Lincoln, they have Wendy (from Wendy's) who about half get right, they have Ronald McDonald who they ***ALL*** get right, and then they have a picture of Jesus Christ that nobody has a clue about. What are we really teaching our most prized possessions, our children? What are they learning through our examples? Is there BodyMindSpirit balance and synergy?

Let's talk briefly about the importance of enjoying our food. Eating is not a burden; it is an adventure! If you are consistently good, reward yourself, splurge a little. Eat some of your favorite dessert or have that candy bar. Take a day and eat anything you desire. If you cook your food, do it in ways that are good to the taste. Eat things that gladden the heart and make you happy to be alive. Some say you can't eat healthy in restaurants. This isn't true; you can usually eat very healthy in most restaurants.

"Eating in a restaurant is often seen as a special time, a chance to indulge yourself. But you can enjoy a meal in virtually any restaurant and still keep healthful eating in mind. Look for menu items that include terms like: Baked, Braised, Broiled, Grilled, Poached, Roasted, Steamed, and stir-fried. Don't hesitate to ask your server or the chef how meals are prepared. Many restaurants will accommodate your request to prepare foods to your liking. Restaurant portions are often larger than serving sizes you prepare at home, so don't feel that you have to eat the whole thing – ask for a takeout container, then enjoy the rest tomorrow."

—American Dietetic Association

One of the saddest parts of the Covid-19 pandemic was the death that swept the world, of course, but from a health educator's perspective it is so sad to lose some of the healthiest restaurant chains in America; Sweet Tomatoes, Fresh Choice, and Soup or Salad. These all-you-can-eat places were great because they generally had really healthy choices; things like spinach, lettuce, beets, radishes, raw carrots and celery, lots of fresh fruit, non-fat and low-calorie dressings, corn, sweet potatoes, peas, fish, baked chicken, and filtered water. Making you hungry? These restaurants made for a great day of healthy and great tasting grub.

A caution here about MSG. MSG is an excitotoxin, a very dangerous chemical. MSG consumption has doubled in every decade in America since 1948.[236] It is in canned soups, packaged meats, cookies, crackers, packaged cereals, potato chips, almost everything with a label. It is disguised many times as Natural Flavors. MSG has significant health risks. If you haven't read much about it do a Google search and read up. MSG is used in virtually every restaurant in America. Sweet Tomatoes said the only food in their restaurant that had MSG was their beets, that were canned, but nothing else has MSG.[237] This is exceptional, for this reason, and because of all the whole food they offered, Sweet Tomatoes was at the top of the list of healthiest restaurants.

One day soon WAVE will have the "WAVE 4 Food" restaurant chain going; creating wonderful foods that taste great and are healthy, in a bright and fun environment, which is reasonably priced. There will be great tasting whole wheat pastas and breads in all their varieties, amazing desserts made with whole grain ingredients; that are sweetened with all natural sweeteners like agave nectar and fructose. Everything will be fresh; no preservatives, no MSG, no harsh chemicals added. There will be fresh fruit, salad, and soup bar. With great variety, depending on what is in season that time of the year. Everything will be organic. It will be a fun place for the whole family...with maybe some challenging games to play before or after food. Maybe even some live entertainment with some of our local talent. Does it sound good and fun? ☺

It's OK to have a cheat meal once in a while. Don't be so uptight that you drive everyone around you crazy. Be consistently good, but don't be a fanatic. You will turn others off instead of turning them on to your healthy lifestyle. Example is the best teacher. If you do have a *cheat meal*, don't do it every week, but rather whenever you feel like you need it. That might be more at first, but when you get in a good routine and find great foods and recipes, you may find that your desire to cheat becomes almost non-existent. Some trainers encourage a cheat day once a week, but this encourages binge eating and deprivation, both of which are *not* good. If your body is craving something, eat it. Most likely your body is telling you it is deficient in certain vitamins or minerals, thus the importance of good nutrition and supplements.

If you have been really strict during the week reward yourself with a meal of fun at the table. If you are consistently good, it won't hurt to periodically do something not so good. Depending on how healthy your nutrition gets, you might find that junk food and candy will not be as appealing as they once were. Like previously mentioned, sometimes it actually becomes sickening; some will throw up from eating greasy food after they have been eating really healthy for a

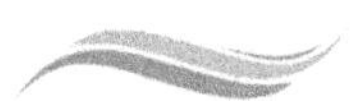

period of time. If you are having strong cravings to binge all the time, you might be too strict too soon. Ease into your healthy lifestyle. If you are craving specific foods, you might not be getting enough nutrition; figure out what your body is telling you. Find out what those favorite spices are at the restaurant, so you can buy them and add them in to your own cooking.

"Salt and pepper aren't your only choices when it comes to spices. Dozens of herbs and spices can provide variety to your cooking, make an old meal new and just add a little fun. Some herbs and spices work better with certain foods, so try the following: bay leaves, basil, thyme and fennel on beef, curry, ginger or sage on chicken; cumin, onion and saffron on rice; and cinnamon, cloves and nutmeg in fruit. Start by adding small amounts of dried herbs at the beginning of cooking. If you enjoy the flavor, add more the next time. When using fresh herbs, add them at the end of cooking and use more than you would for dried, since fresh herbs aren't as strong. Experimenting with herbs and spices can give your food a new twist."

—American Dietetic Association

Compliment your wife, mother, husband, or father on their cooking, so it makes it more enjoyable for them to cook.

"There is no spectacle on earth more appealing than that of a beautiful woman in the act of cooking dinner for someone she loves."

—Thomas Wolfe

Discuss your favorite dishes over the dinner table so people know what you like. Help in the kitchen with the dishes afterward, so it is not such a burden to cook. Maybe whoever cooks gets to relax while the others do the dishes, or maybe everyone cooks and cleans up together?

Build your own favorite recipes. There are thousands of recipes on the WAVE website, wave4life.com Login and go to the online

magazine. You will find many great recipes and instructions on how to make them. When you eat something really good find out who made it and ask them for the recipe. It will amaze you how quickly you can build up your own favorite recipe book. If there are unhealthy additives, substitute healthy ones. You usually don't need to follow the recipe exactly to make it good; use a healthy oil like avocado oil instead of butter, use fructose or agave nectar instead of sugar. There is usually always something that tastes just as good, maybe even better, without all the animal fat (saturated fat) or large amounts of processed sugar. Be creative. Have fun parties and get-togethers, with healthy food. Have everyone bring their favorite dish or dessert. Give prizes out for the best tasting dish, the healthiest dish, etc.

"Many people equate 'healthy eating' with 'having no choices' or 'tastes bad.' If that describes you, spice up your menu with ethnic cuisine. If you're hesitant to try ethnic cooking, start slowly. Work a few new foods into your repertoire or just season familiar dishes differently. Try: Tabouli, dolmas, baklava and falafel (Greek); Burritos, enchiladas, gazpacho and flan (Mexican); Spring rolls, stir-fried tofu and pad Thai (Thai); Tandoori chicken, lentil dishes and naan (Indian). If you find you're enjoying ethnic foods, slowly add more choices to your meal planning and sample more options when dining out. And don't be afraid to ask questions about ingredients or preparation."

—American Dietetic Association

Original Fast Foods, is a great book about nutrition; the authors are Jim and Colleen Simmons.[238] Jim was raised on a farm in Idaho, his dad was a doctor, and his mom was a nutritionist. Colleen's dad worked for General Mills. So, when they got married and started raising a family, they had a pretty typical America nutrition program with lots of meat and dairy, and lots of processed food. Jim was healthy for a time but then went through a period of 10 years where he was barely able to go to work and perform his normal duties. He visited doctor after doctor trying to figure out what the problem was.

Eventually he went to the Lord in prayer and fasting asking for help to figure out what was the problem and how to get rid of it. He started a raw nutrition program and within 6 months his health was completely restored. He then went on to introduce his family to a nutrition program that centers on fruits, vegetables, whole grains, legumes, nuts, and seeds, then eventually wrote a book about his experience. In his book he and his wife list *hundreds of recipes* that are loved by all 10 of his kids, yes, he really has 10. This book is great for anyone who is suffering from poor health or just wants to look and feel better. Go to originalfastfoods.com to purchase the book and learn more.

Let's talk for a moment about dinnertime. What if we have family time around the dinner table so everyone looks forward to dinner, or breakfast? The average American child gets 7-11 minutes of conversation a day with their parents.[239] But the average American child watches TV 4 hours a day.[240] Who is really raising our children? *What If...*we *turn off the TV and get to know our family?* Don't let the kids eat and run away from the table. Make it a time of sharing, caring and love. Start the meal with a prayer of thanksgiving; this will build gratitude in the hearts of your children and bring more of God's blessing into your lives. Maybe ask each child to share what they did for someone else that day. Have the kids help clean up after the meal, so they get in the habit, and when they are older it will just be something they do automatically. Your children's spouse will love you for it. Kids love to work by the side of an adult. Teach the children how to cook. Ask them what they like. Make eating time enjoyable and memorable, not a chore.

When talking about Words of Wisdom it's important to mention the importance of ***WATER.*** If people live by the other principles taught here, like exercise, they most likely will get all the water they need. Most of our bodies are made out of water. It is the most important thing we can take into our bodies. We can live for a long time without food or exercise, but not long without water. How much

do you need every day? Do you remember what Dr. Lorraine Day tells us? ***Ten glasses*** of water per day.[241] You will get a lot of water in food like fruits that are mostly water; another reason why fruit is so important. A lot of vegetables also have lots of water. Of course, water is all water. ☺ Stay away from the pop, the carbonation actually dehydrates you, drink water not soda.[242]

Some carry a big water jug wherever they go, so they remember to drink. Here's a little secret that works, *EXERCISE.* If you exercise you will naturally drink all the water you need. You will not have to force yourself to drink. Drink alkaline water, we will talk more about this soon.

Dehydration is linked to as many diseases as is stress. The list is exhaustive: Bad backs, diabetes, high blood pressure, obesity, heart disease, headaches, multiple sclerosis, asthma, nausea...the list goes on and on.[243] If you exercise and drink water you will be a lot healthier, and avoid many of the diseases that afflict us.

These are some words of wisdom. There are so many more. Please see the Appendix or the WAVE website, wave4life.com for references of good reading material. Be wise and learn from words of wisdom and truth.

QUESTION EVERYTHING?
MOM,
SO WE CAN CHEAT IN
EATING SOMETIMES?
QETommy.com

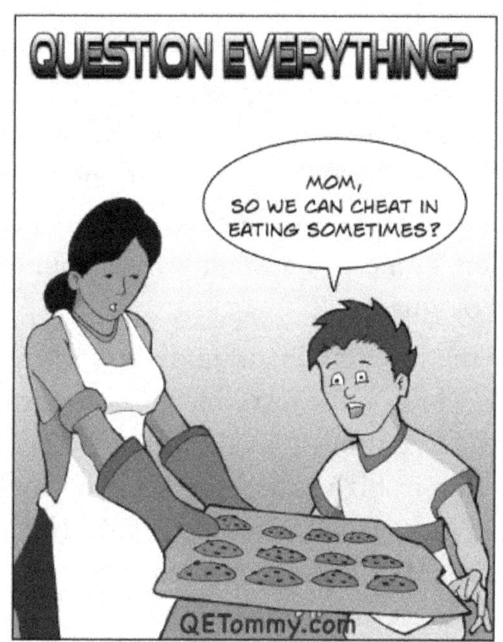

PRINCIPLE #6
Eat Foods Low On The Glycemic Index
To keep your body fat low and your energy high

The Glycemic Index ranks carbohydrates by how quickly they are broken down into *glucose*.[244] All food that is used as energy is eventually broken down into glucose. Glucose is our body's usable source of energy.[245] Sugar is broken down immediately. On a scale of 0-100, sugar ranks 100. When you take in large quantities of sugar, your blood sugar level rises quickly. This is a dangerous situation for your body to be in so your pancreas releases *insulin*. Insulin does 2 basic things: it lowers your blood sugar, and it pulls fat to your fat stores.[246] This is why when you eat sugary breakfast cereals, or a candy bar, you might feel an instant surge of energy, but then you hit

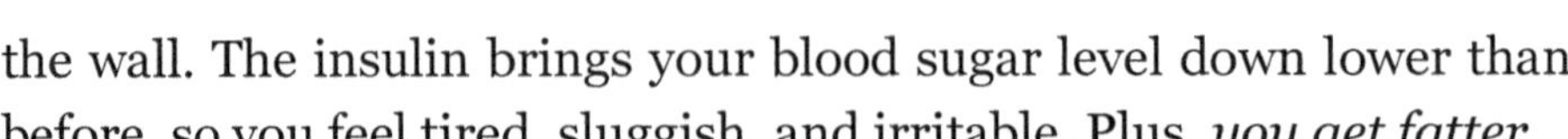

the wall. The insulin brings your blood sugar level down lower than before, so you feel tired, sluggish, and irritable. Plus, *you get fatter*.

When we eat foods low on the glycemic index *glucagon* is released not insulin.[247] Glucagon has about the opposite effect as insulin.[248] It helps keep blood sugar levels constant and pulls fat out of your fat stores. You lose body fat and have consistent energy levels with no mood swings. Here's an easy question, which would you rather have released, insulin or glucagon?

This is why the low carbohydrate diets work. When people eat foods that are very low on the glycemic index, things like meat, fats, vegetables and water, glucagon is released, not insulin. Even though their diet is likely very high in fat, the fat is not pulled to their fat stores, so people can actually lose body fat. Their inward health (triglycerides, LDL, HDL) also improves much of the time, which is amazing considering all the fat that they're eating.[249] The diet (4-letter word) works. But what about the negative affects? Not many antioxidants, too much meat, too much fat, low energy, and poor long-term health. Wouldn't it be better to just follow these 7 Principles of Healthy Nutrition and achieve all the beneficial results and none of the bad?

The goal is to have adequate blood sugar levels throughout the day so you have consistent energy and your blood sugar is never spiked. You can do this by eating regularly (constant nourishment), and by eating foods *low* on the glycemic index. Most hypoglycemic people are forced to eat this way, and most have very low body fat. They eat small meals often and usually stay away from the high glycemic foods.

The absolute worst combination of foods you can eat is a high glycemic food and a high fat food, something like processed chocolate.[250] The sugar in the chocolate raises your blood sugar, *insulin* is released, and it lowers your blood sugar. Then the insulin takes the fat in the chocolate and brings it to your fat stores...you get *fatter*. Even worse is something with a lot of fat in it, something with

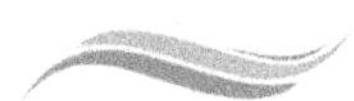

maybe peanut butter in it. Peanuts are pretty nutritious. They are high in protein and most of the fats are good fats—fats our bodies need at every meal; but with sugar, not a good combination. Now, a little chocolate isn't going to hurt anyone. If you are consistently good, it doesn't hurt to splurge a little. But if you are consistently bad, watch out!

It is not the chocolate that is bad, chocolate it is actually good for us. The ORAC (antioxidant) value in chocolate is one of the highest of any food; it is the man-made sugar and fat in it that makes it so bad.[251] There is good tasting healthy chocolate out there in the marketplace; you just have to search for it. WAVE will produce this healthy chocolate one day; keep your eye out for it. ☺

What about bread and pasta? White bread and white pasta give bread & pasta a bad name. White bread and white pasta have a glycemic index of about 70 or higher, depending on how processed (stripped of nutrients) the white flour is.[252] Whole wheat bread & pasta have glycemic indexes of about 50; usually the darker it is the lower glycemic index it has. 50 is not much higher than the low glycemic index foods like meat and dairy, which are generally in the 30-40 range.[253] Buy the whole wheat breads & pasta for your family. Once you eat whole grains for a period of time you will likely lose your desire for white breads & pasta. Except for maybe sour dough, white bread and pasta will lack taste, and you know it lacks nutrition. This is one thing WAVE will do with our chain of restaurants, serve great tasting whole wheat bread & pasta...WAVE 4 Food, look for it!

Most vegetables are low on the glycemic index, except for a few starchy vegetables like carrots (80) and peas and corn (about 60).[254] Fruits are generally pretty low, especially the northern fruits (orange, berries, apple). Equatorial fruits (banana, mango, papaya) tend to be a bit higher. Some people ask, why aren't fruits high, they have a lot of sugar in them? Yes, but mostly fructose ("fruit sugar"), which has a glycemic index of about 20.[255] Blessed are the children that are raised

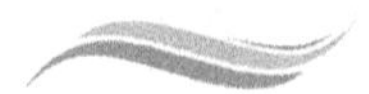

with fruit instead of sugar around the house. When the child matures, they will love fruit and likely be a lot healthier than kids that were raised on sugar.

"Train up a child in the way he should go and when he is old, he will not depart from it."

—Proverbs 22:6

For a more extensive list of low, medium, and high glycemic index foods look online.

Since some foods are so high on the glycemic index should we avoid them completely or just eat less of them? It isn't necessary to cut anything completely out of your nutrition program (except maybe tobacco), just use caution. Carrots, for instance, are very high, but you need them for how jam-packed they are with nutrients such as vitamin A, especially if you eat them raw. Just be careful not to eat them with a bunch of fat.

Another important point is when you eat foods in combination with one another, the glycemic index changes. If you mix a carrot (glycemic index of 80) with fruit or another vegetable that has a glycemic index of 30, the result might be a food that has a glycemic index of 50. Some take this and create the philosophy that it really doesn't do any good to worry about high vs. low glycemic index foods, because in combination they all change. Yes, but it makes sense that if you generally choose foods low on the glycemic index, the overall value will turn out low, as will the opposite be true.

As we talk about low glycemic index foods, it might be helpful to take a look at the government's recommendations of the foods they suggest in the Food Pyramid, so we can get a clearer picture of the foods that are most important in our daily nutrition.

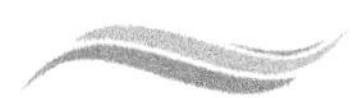

"You can make healthy food choices and enjoy physical activity most days of the week. If you're ready to start a new health regimen, first disregard any diet that promises to be the answer to all your weight loss needs or guarantees success. Forget diets that require you to avoid entire food groups or make claims about the magic of certain foods. Write down what you are eating, compare your intake to the Food Guide Pyramid and use the results to outline a plan for change. Contact dietetics professional for help in constructing a plan that is right for you."

—American Dietetic Association

So, let's take this counsel to heart and make the governments Food Pyramid even healthier. Included in the Appendix is a weeks' worth of recording pages for your nutrition; when you write everything down that you eat it will focus your mind on improvement. This process of writing down everything you're eating is as motivating as getting your body fat measured. You will get disgusted, motivated, frustrated, you will get competitive with your old self, and others, and you will be more apt to make the necessary changes to live a healthier, happier life. Just follow the instructions in the Appendix and see how you come out. Maybe you will be one of those who surprise yourself? If so, hat's off to you.

Government Pyramid GOOD	WAVE Pyramid BETTER YET
Fats and Sweets Sparingly	Animal Fats Sweets Sparingly
2-3 Milk, Yogurt, & Cheese	1-2 *Organic* Soy Milk, Rice Milk 0-1 *Organic* Non-Fat Milk, Yogurt, or Cheese
2-3 Meat, Poultry, Fish, Dry Beans, Eggs and Nuts	2-3 *Organic* Beans, Nuts & Seeds 0-1 *Organic* Meat, Poultry, Fish, Egg
2-4 Fruit	2-5 *Organic Fruit* (Instead of sugar)
3-5 Vegetables	3-6 *Organic* Vegetables (Preferably raw or steamed)
6-11 Servings of Bread Cereal, Pasta & Rice	4-6 Servings of *Organic* Whole Wheat Bread, Pasta & Rice

Here are the details of some changes to the Food Pyramid to make it even healthier. Let's start at the bottom and work our way up.

6-11 Servings of Bread, Cereal, Pasta, and Rice

Better Yet:

4-6 Servings of Organic Whole Wheat & Whole Grains (Bread, Pasta, Cereal), and Rice

Organic food is generally going to be better than regular grocery store food, although most regular grocery stores now have organic food also. This might not have been true 30 years ago, but it is today. Organic food generally has more nutrition, has less of the harsh chemicals (pesticides & preservatives), and is usually processed less than the regular store-bought varieties.[256] A peer-reviewed University of Washington study found that children who consumed conventional foods had six to nine times more pesticide residues in their bodies than children who consumed organic foods.[257]

With organic meat, the animal was usually free roaming and grain fed. It is also usually steroid and growth hormone free. The organic varieties may not be as big and pretty, but it should taste better and be much better for you. The term *usually* is used because sometimes the organic food isn't much different than the regular grocery store food. Become proficient at reading labels, or better yet don't buy anything with a label on it. Get in the habit of asking knowledgeable people who work in the health food stores about the food. One of the big objections to organic food is the cost. If you look for things on sale, or buy directly from the farmer, you will eliminate much of the extra cost. Or better yet, grow your own, which is basically free!

The best thing you can do is become informed; know where your food is coming from, what the farmers use in the soils, and how long they rest the soils. Again, it is best to grow your own; then you know exactly what you are getting. You can pick the food when it is ripe and ready which will allow the food to be as nutritious as possible. It is also great for kids to see the process of growing food; it helps them appreciate the wonderful world we live in. Obviously, this isn't always possible, especially in the cities, but it eliminates all the guess work.

Whole grains are always better than the bleached flour with nutrients added back in. Not that supplements aren't important, but your body can assimilate (use) the nutrients in *whole food* much better than man-made nutrients added in after processing. As mentioned earlier, there is a lot more nutrition in whole food than in supplements. Less processing and less man-made chemicals create better food. When food is processed it is generally heated and toxic chemicals are added in to preserve the food's freshness for shelf life at the grocery store.

The closer you can get to Mother Earth the better. Of course, much of the processing and preservatives are necessary to ensure the safety of the food we eat. This is why raw food or homegrown food is best; you likely won't use all the harsh pesticides and preservatives, and you can control the heating that destroys much of the nutritional value. Plus, your soil will likely be healthier than other soils; if you let it rest (don't plant in it over and over) and take care to make it nutritious by adding healthy fertilizers. Just be conscious of the fact that the more natural a food can be, considering safety, the better.

Unless you are an athlete in training 4-6 servings of grains are sufficient; eat more nutrient dense foods like vegetables and fruit.

3-5 Vegetables

Better Yet:

3-6 *Organic* Vegetables (Preferably raw or steamed)

If possible, buy organic or grow your own. As stated above, cooking will destroy much of the nutritional value - the less cooking, processing, preservatives, the better. Raw fruits and vegetables are best; be cautious with some raw food recipes, they are generally more nutritious but make sure they are safe. Steaming is great if you like the vegetables soft. Cooking them in water, especially at high temperatures, destroys many of the nutrients, and transfers many of the other nutrients to the cooking water.[258]

2-4 Fruit

Better Yet:

2-5 *Organic* Fruit (Instead of sugar)

If possible, buy organic or grow your own. Fruit is a great substitute for sugar. It is said that if you take an infant just able to eat and place before them candy, meat, fruit, and vegetables, they will choose the *fruit*; so many of our likes and dislikes are conditioned behaviors.[259]

2-3 Meat, Poultry, Fish, Dry Beans, Eggs and Nuts

Better Yet:

1-2 Organic Beans, Nuts & Seeds/ 0-1 Organic Meat, Poultry, Fish, Eggs

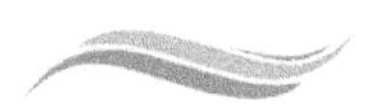

Buy organic or grow your own. Beans and brown or wild rice are a great combination food that has lots of complex carbohydrates and protein. What a great combination instead of meat. It is so much easier on our body to digest, and it takes so much less of our earth's resources to create it. Nuts are great too. Use some caution with nuts because they have a lot of fat, but it's mostly the good kind of fat. Remember to avoid eating a lot of fat and sugar together.

Eat meat *sparingly* and with *thanksgiving*. Enjoy the wonderful flavor. It's best to cook it outside on a grill so most of the fat drips out, and that outdoor grilled taste is *so* good. Egg Beaters (eggs without the yolk) are best, all the protein from real eggs, but no cholesterol or animal fat. White meat is likely better than red meat; it has less fat and is not as tough, thus easier for your body to digest. Fish is likely better than white meat. It generally has less fat and is softer, thus easier for your body to digest. But watch the mercury levels in fish.

"Humans are exposed to methyl mercury primarily through eating fish. So widespread has this problem become that one out of every six women of childbearing age in the United States today has blood mercury concentrations high enough to damage a developing fetus. This means that 630,000 of the four million babies born in the United States each year are likely to experience some level of neurological damage because of exposure to hazardous mercury levels in the womb."[260]

—John Robbins

Again, buy the organic varieties or hunt your own; looks for animals that are generally grain fed, free roaming, steroid, growth hormone, and mercury free - much better for you.

2-3 Milk, Yogurt, and Cheese

Better Yet:

1-2 Organic Soy Milk, Rice Milk/ 0-1 Organic Non-Fat Milk, Yogurt and Cheese

Buy organic or grow your own. Dairy is best viewed as dessert, or something to help us create more flavor in our food. It is high in protein, but most is hard for our bodies to digest. Up to 70% of the world's population does not produce enough of the enzyme lactase, which is responsible for the digestion of lactose, and therefore has some degree of lactose intolerance. This should tell us something![261]

Milk and dairy products are also high in hormones, bacteria, and many other not so appealing things. Store bought milk has over 50 hormones in it, is it any wonder some of our kids are entering puberty now at 12, 10 and even 8 or less?[262] Goat's milk is better than cow's milk.[263] It's more nutritious and the protein is easier for our body to process. Even raw cow's milk that looks and tastes like cream and is higher in fat is probably better than the low-fat pasteurized & homogenized variety in the grocery store. It is more nutritious and has all the enzymes that help break down all the fat that is in it.

Whole milk in the grocery store is 49% fat.[264] It's the kind of fat our bodies do not need – animal fat (mostly saturated fat). If you insist on drinking milk, or can't live without it on your breakfast cereal, get the raw or non-fat variety. Of course, you should be cautious of dairy that is raw. It's more nutritious but make sure it's safe. A better choice than cow or goat milk might be soy, almond, or rice milk. But be careful of GMO (Genetically modified) products, and those with lots of other added ingredients. Low-fat and non-fat products are sometimes better, sometimes worse, than more natural products. They're high in protein and have no animal products. They're vegetables and grains. For some it might get some getting used to, but they really taste good, better than milk once you get used to them. But some are high in added sugar, so read the labels; they list ingredients in the order of quantity, if sugar is high on the list watch out.

Many people use the calcium excuse for milk. The fact is that most people get more than enough calcium in their daily nutrition.

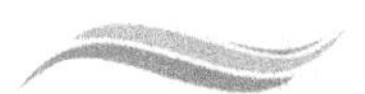

According to Dr. Lorraine Day, the cause of osteoporosis is ***not*** too little calcium, rather:

1. Too much animal protein.[265] To add to this here's a second thing just as important:
2. Not enough exercise.

Osteoporosis is highest in the countries (like America) that have the highest animal product consumption.[266] When you eat a lot of animal protein your blood acid levels rise, because these foods are acidic, and in order to neutralize this dangerous condition your body leaches calcium from your bones. There is *lots* of documentation (peer reviewed medical journals) to substantiate this fact.[267]

Another cause of osteoporosis is lack of exercise.[268] When you put pressure on your bones through exercise, they absorb the calcium in your nutrition. If we eat nutritious fruits, vegetables, and whole grains we will get more than enough calcium in our nutrition to supply for our needs, and if we exercise our bones will absorb the needed calcium we consume. It is so simple, yet most have no idea what causes osteoporosis, or how to prevent or reverse the problem. Why? Because the meat and dairy industries want to sell us animal products.

We have been told that milk and dairy products build strong bones, when in fact they do just the opposite.[269] We have been lied to for years. *Fruits, vegetables, whole grains, and exercise* are the things that do a body good.

When you use cheese, use the low-fat or non-fat varieties. Splurge sometimes with some ice cream of your favorite variety, or try some yogurt. But be cautious with all meat and dairy products.

Fats and Sweets Sparingly

Better Yet:

Animal Fats and Sweets Sparingly

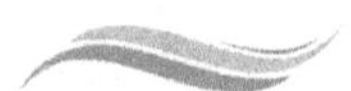

Your body needs fat at every meal, the vegetable fats, not the animal fats. So, cook with avocado oil, or virgin olive oil. But remember that oils are very high in fat, and do not have much nutrition per calorie (very low on the Nutrient Density Chart). Olive oil's nutrition can be lost when heated to high temperatures. Many people think we need oils or fish to get our Omega-3 fatty acids, but you can get plenty of them from greens, soybeans, nuts and seeds.[270] It's ok to eat some sugar, but the organic whole cane variety is a lot better for you than the processed white sugar. Just be careful before meals.

Sugar will spoil your appetite, boost your blood sugar levels, cause insulin to be released, and make you fat. When you are consistently bad is when you will have problems. Real sugar (from the earth) is much better than the man-made chemicals used for sweeteners. NutraSweet (aspartame) is bad news, avoid it. It accounts for 75% of all the adverse reactions of food additives that is reported to the FDA.[271] Our government tells pilots and pregnant women to avoid even 1 stick of chewing gum with NutraSweet, so should you![272]

Agave nectar from cactus is a great sweetener for cooking. Stevia is a plant and has been used as a sweetener for hundreds of years in South America. It is being increasingly used in Japan but received a bad rap from the FDA from a flawed study in 1991, that has since been

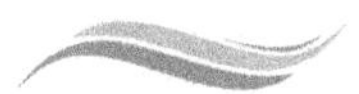

discredited.[273] It is virtually non-caloric and has proven nutritional benefits.

"Resolve to do something you really can carry out. Don't resolve to completely give up certain foods that you enjoy or vow to achieve unrealistic levels of exercise. If you fall short of unreasonable goals, you'll feel like you've failed when that's not actually the case. Resolve to develop an eating and exercise plan that you can follow. Assess your eating habits, including what and how much you eat. Check your list against the Food Guide Pyramid to determine where you need to make changes. Then, make a plan that involves one small change per week. Switch from whole milk to two percent or add one serving of fruit or vegetables to your diet each day, gradually working up to at least five a day. Plan and make achievable changes in your eating plan and levels of physical activity."

—American Dietetic Association

Good advice. Complete the Nutritional Analysis in the Appendix and hire one of our registered dieticians at wave4life.com if you need help following this counsel.

QUESTION EVERYTHING?
PIRATE ORR, HAVE YOU TRIED EATING MORE FRUITS AND VEGETABLES?
QETommy.com

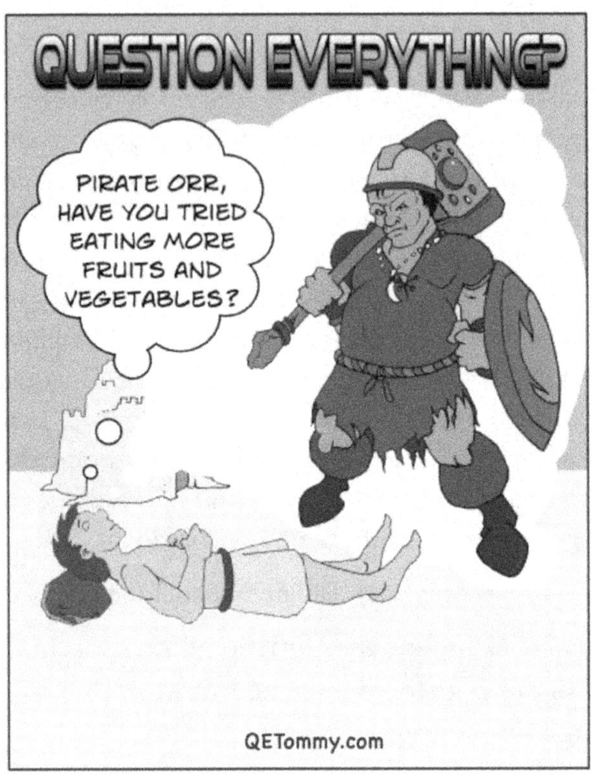

PRINCIPLE #7
Use A BodyMindSpirit Approach To Your Nutrition

Anything less and you go in circles

Your time and attention as you've read through these principles of healthy nutrition is appreciated. Hopefully you have learned some things that you might not have considered before, that will help your life a healthier, happier life.

Many of our physical ailments can be reversed with good nutrition.

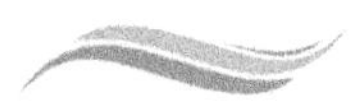

Remember that it is not the food, exercise or supplement that is curing the disease; rather you are giving your body the nutrition it needs to naturally heal itself.

Remember also that we are more than just body, we are BodyMindSpirit, and if you or someone you love is afflicted in any way physically, it might be the mind or spirit that is suffering but manifesting the problem through the body.

YOU can help to make America, and the rest of the world, a healthier and happier place. Maybe you are someone who has a lot of influence and believes in what you read here, please come help, there's plenty to do. Maybe you know someone that has a lot of influence and would possibly like to help, maybe give them this book, and encourage them read it. Maybe you have a firm belief in God and prayer. If so, your prayers are sincerely appreciated. Thank you in advance for all you do.

Maybe you are a mother raising beautiful children. By setting a good example for your children you are influencing their lives, and all your future posterity, you are to be saluted for your efforts, thank you for being such a great teacher and former of lives!

Maybe you are nobody significant, just a common person with a simple life, but by doing something for someone else that is good and right and kind, like the movie, *Pay It Forward*; your simple acts of kindness will start a cycle of goodness that never stops, and ends up blessing thousands of lives.

You are a begotten son or daughter of God. You have more potential, influence, intelligence and goodness within you than you could ever imagine. You are to be honored for all you do to better your life and our world.

May you find this greatness and be all that you can be. God bless you toward this end.

QUESTION EVERYTHING?
MR. PHOENIX, DID YOUR DAD MAKE YOU GET HAIR CUTS?
QETommy.com

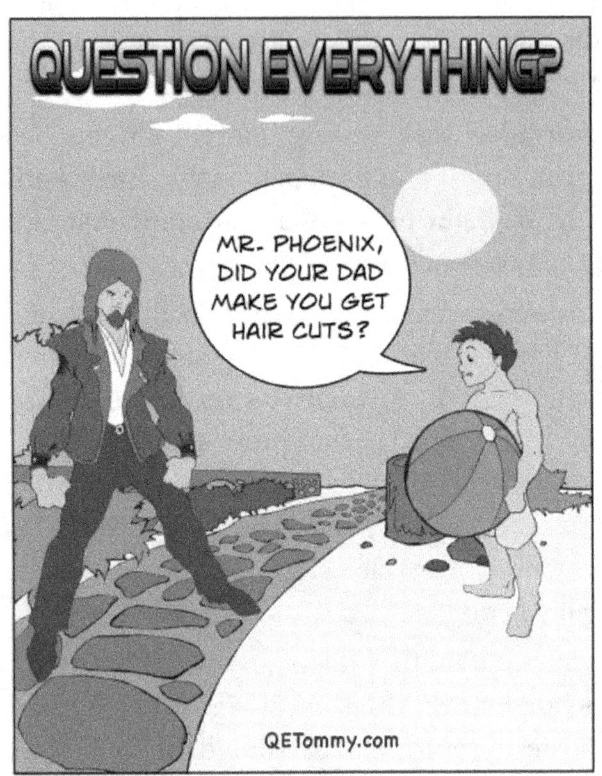

7 PRINCIPLES OF A HEALTHY MIND

"I had many problems in my life, most of which never happened."

—Mark Twain

INTRODUCTION

The purpose of the 7 Principles of a Healthy Mind is to help you live a healthy, happy, and productive life.

Just like a healthy body, a healthy mind is something we *create*. Yes, some people are born into situations that are more conducive to a healthy mind than others, but ultimately it is up to us to be happy, have joy, overcome our circumstances, and rise above it all. Herein lies the purpose of this earthy life, not to be products of our environment or circumstances, but rather to create a healthy, happy, productive life. Within us all lies true greatness.

This discussion will call upon the words of wise men and women throughout the ages. The objective is to teach correct principles of healthy living, and appeal to most everyone of every faith and belief system. Sometimes the words of truth are hard for people to swallow, because if they accept them as truth they might need to change, and many do not want to change.

"Men often stumble over the truth, but most pick themselves up and hurry on as if nothing had happened"

—Winston Churchill

The position of this book is not one of force or coercion, but rather freedom of thought and expression, and a deep respect for all people, and all belief systems. For this reason, this discussion will focus upon the thoughts and words of wise men and women throughout the ages. But remember, the objective is to teach truth, and our minds and spirits are connected and related.

QUESTION EVERYTHING?
DAVID,
HOW COME KIDS
LAUGH SO MUCH
MORE THAN
ADULTS?
QETommy.com

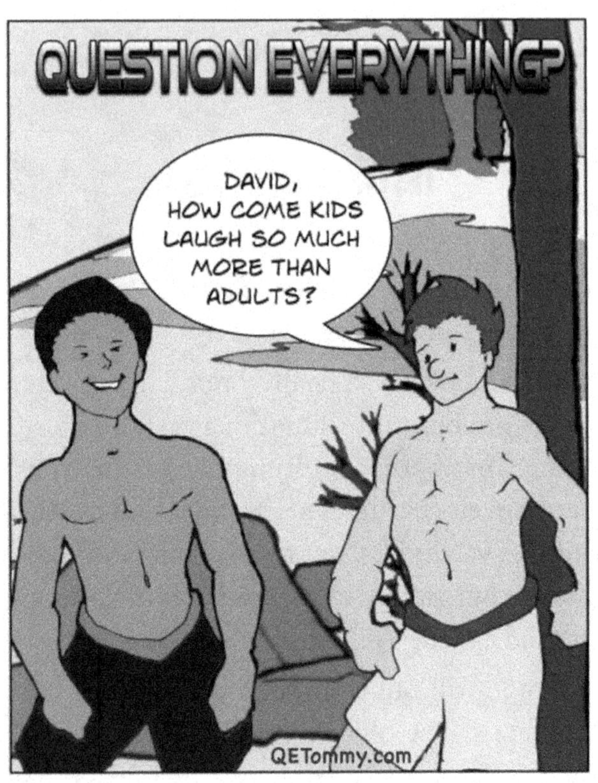

PRINCIPLE #1
Think And Grow Rich

You are what you think about

"We are what we repeatedly do.
Excellence, then, is not an act, but a habit."

—Aristotle

It has been said a million times because it is true; you are the sum total of all your thoughts. If you want to change yourself, your environment or circumstances in life, change what you think about.

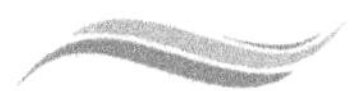

If you want to be a positive person, think positive thoughts; if you want to be a negative person, think negative thoughts. If you want to better your situation in life, think about being in that situation where you already have what you desire...eventually you will achieve what you think about.

"The quality of a person's life is in direct proportion to their commitment to excellence, regardless of their chosen field of endeavor."

—Vince Lombardi

If this is true, then why is anyone negative, poor, destitute, or in an environment or circumstances that are lacking? Why would we not all be committed to this excellence? None of us really want the bad things in life. It can be very difficult to change our thinking, thus our environment. Some people just go with the flow and live out their lives in mediocrity. Some may believe that they don't have much control over their environment or circumstances in life. Others may focus on things they think will bring them happiness and satisfaction, but many times in reality these are counterfeits.

You deserve the best, don't settle for less.[274] Don't be one of those who has true joy and happiness staring them right in the face, but do not recognize it because they are looking in the wrong places, and are focused on the wrong objectives. Don't let the world tell you what will make you happy. You figure it out, and if that doesn't sit well with everyone around you, do not be kept from your dream. Your voice and vision should be your guiding force. Not all the other voices around you.

As you learn to navigate toward your greatest health and happiness you'll realize it's important to forge a new plan based on your own research and commitment to excellence. Don't give into old ways or ideas just because it is what you were taught by parents, friends, teachers, someone in your environment. Rise above the world

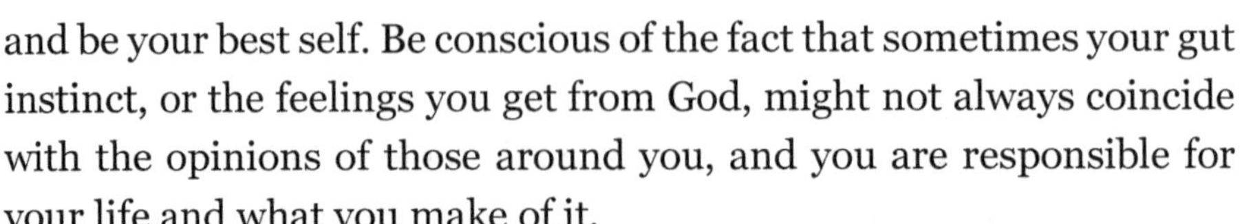

and be your best self. Be conscious of the fact that sometimes your gut instinct, or the feelings you get from God, might not always coincide with the opinions of those around you, and you are responsible for your life and what you make of it.

Are you a winner or a loser? It's up to you. We all have all the potential in the world, yet we often waste it and sell it for a mess of pottage, or for a handful of coins...so sad.[275]

"Whatever the mind of man can conceive and believe, it can achieve."

—Napoleon Hill

Will we continue to let our circumstances rule our life? Or will we take charge, arise from the dust, and do what we are capable of doing? Life can be heaven on earth, but it must first begin with what we think about.

When our lives are drawing to a close do, we go to our graves thinking about what might have been, or do we think more along the lines of a life of no regrets, that we became all that we could be? It is up to us. We are the creators of our own destinies, the masters of our own souls. We alone are responsible for our circumstances and positions in life...so, how do we rise above it all, not give in to our environments or circumstances, live a life of no regrets, and become all that we are capable of becoming? Through God's help we can *focus and control our thoughts.*

In Napoleon Hill's classic book, *Think and Grow Rich,* he outlines a system to change our thoughts, thus our environment.[276] This book is great for anyone who is not satisfied with where they are in life; hopefully all of us want to improve. A few short words here can summarize his thoughts, but to get a real flavor of his writing you must get a copy of his book and read it again and again until it really sinks in...it is said that we need to read or hear something about *16 times* to really comprehend what is being said.[277] Of all the things

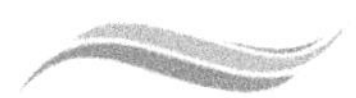

to learn about in this world isn't it most important to learn about who we really are, what we can become, and how to overcome our circumstances in life and be all that we can be?

So much precious time in life is wasted. How many hours are spent watching mediocre entertainment on TV, reading books that are entertaining but offer no real value, mess around on the Internet, or spend countless hours with video games...all the while we could be focused on developing our talents, seeking the truth and wisdom all around us, learning how to be leaders, masters of our own souls and destinies, and creators of our own joy and happiness.

So, if we are the sum total of all our thoughts, and they really do shape who we are and what we accomplish in life, how do we control them and focus them on what we want in life? In the great book, *The Secret*, it is said that we have about 60,000 thoughts a day, and the good news is that a positive thought is 100 times more powerful than a negative one. The authors say that one of the best ways to control our thoughts is to attach emotion with the thoughts we desire the most, then they are burned into our minds and hearts, and we remember them and tend to automatically focus on them the most.[278] Then the *law of attraction* (like attracts like) comes into play and we get what we think about and desire the most.[279] If we attach emotion to our positive thoughts the power in our lives will increase.

A good way to help us focus on positive, faithful, and grateful thoughts is through "faithful affirmations" that we write down and read daily, or maybe a couple times a week. Take a day and write down a few of them, maybe 5-20, and when you accomplish one either attach a gratitude-type statement to it and keep it, or cross it off and replace it with another. Don't make it too cumbersome, otherwise you might not do it regularly or often enough to make a difference. Read them with emotion and out loud if possible. An example might be, "I am so thankful that I am a happy and joyful person." If you read these in the morning, it will help you get your day off to a great start. If you

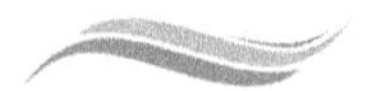

say them at night, it will put you into a grateful and positive state of mind before you go to sleep. If you say them when discouraged it will help you realize how blessed you really are.

Another thing that will help you in your life is training the subconscious mind, just like you do your conscious mind, to think the thoughts you want to focus on, so you bring them to pass.

"You attract to you the predominant thoughts that
you're holding in your awareness,
whether those thoughts are conscious or unconscious."

—Michael Bernard Beckwith

Athletes hear about this all the time. This is why visualization is so important. Our subconscious mind cannot tell the difference between an actual event and one made up in our mind, so if we visualize success in our mind, it helps create that success in real life.[280] Each of us was endowed with more infinite possibilities and the ability to manifest those possibilities through the power of our own minds through proper visualization.

Another thing *The Secret* talks a lot about is the importance of focusing on what want, not what we don't want.[281]

Most people are habitually thinking about what they don't want. If we say, 'I don't want to be poor', the law of attraction reads it as, 'I want to be poor', if we say, 'I don't want to be lonely and unloved', the law of attraction reads it as, 'I want to be lonely and unloved.'Why would this be true? Because whatever it is that you are focusing on, even if it is not what you want, you are still thinking about it and thus it will come to pass. It has been said again and again that what you resist persists.

Athletes use these techniques a lot. It is easy to say, "I don't want to miss this putt, I have so much riding on it, I just don't want to miss it!" It's so much better to say, "I can make this putt", or "I have

confidence that I will make this putt." It makes a lot of sense that if we focus on what we want we will be more likely to get it.

It is very easy to get discouraged or upset when you are playing poorly. In most sports this will kill you. Maybe in something like football negative emotions can help, but in most sports tension and frustration will create a slower and less effective athlete.[282] When you make a bad shot or play poorly do not give it any emotion, hardly acknowledge it. This might take some time to master. It is a matter of changing our thought process and realizing that negative thoughts rarely help. You might need to learn something from your poor performance, but do not give it emotion, because if you do it will stick with you a lot longer and affect subsequent thoughts, and thus your performance will not be as good. When you make those amazing plays or shots, *celebrate*. Maybe even write the positive experiences down after you play or practice so you remember them. Play them often in your mind every day. The great golfer Fred Couples does this before every shot he makes. He will think about the best shot he has ever made that is like the one he is just about to hit.[283]

In Johnny Millers book, *I Call the Shots*, he talks about playing with Jack Nicklaus and how he has never heard him get upset with himself over a bad shot. He said the only thing he ever heard him say was, "Oh Jack", once when he made a bad shot.[284] There is another great story about Jack Nicklaus that one of the premiere sport psychologists in golf right now, Bob Rotella, relates in his book, *Putting Out of Your Mind*. Bob tells about a friend of his that said Jack made the comment on air one day that he has never missed a short putt in a critical situation in tournament play. Bob's friend said this isn't true, that he saw Jack miss a really short putt just a couple weeks before he said this in the final round of a tournament. He went on to say that he could get a copy of that tournament on tape and the putt that Jack missed and show it to Bob, to prove that Jack was wrong, that he just missed one a few days before he said this.

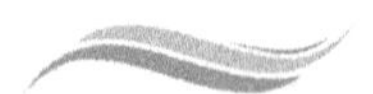

Bob asked his friend what his handicap is. His friend responded that it was something like 15. For those of you who are not golfers, a 15 handicap means you are an average of about 15 shots over par every time you play a round (18 holes) of golf. Bob then said to his friend (paraphrasing), "Jack shoots below par; who do you think is better for people to emulate, someone like Jack that doesn't remember his mistakes and shoots below par, or someone like you that remembers them but shoots 15 shots above par?" (*Putting Out of Your Mind*, p.123)

There is a reason why golfers are so calm; you don't often see the guys that rap their clubs around trees being successful on the PGA Tour. Just like life in general, golf is a mental game, and the better you get at controlling your thoughts, the better golfer you will be. In his younger years Tiger did get very emotional when he missed his shots, and he often still does, but it is said that when he is done being upset, he has an amazing ability to put it behind him and not let it carry over into subsequent shots. Maybe this is a big reason why he's one of the best that's ever been? Can you remember seeing him celebrate his victories? They show them over and over again on TV.

How does all this relate to you? Live your life like Jack Nicklaus does on the golf course. Put the mistakes and bad shots behind you. Do not think about them again unless there is something to be learned by them. Do not give them any emotion, so they do not stick with your conscious or subconscious mind, and therefore you will not attract bad things to your life. Focus on the positive and forget about the negative and attach emotion and gratitude to the good things in life. Through training our mind, we can come to the realization that we have no limits.

Let's talk for a moment about some of the other qualities that determine our success in life. A group of 200 executives were asked what makes a person successful. 80% listed enthusiasm as the most important quality.

Get excited about your life!

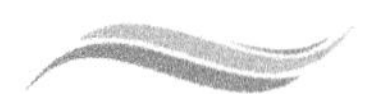

Find that person or whatever it is that will make you enthusiastic about life. Don't leave things to chance and figure you have no control over your life. You are in control. Pray to God for His help then go to work.

Life can be heaven or hell; it's mostly what we make of it. Nobody can destroy our happiness. This can be a hard principle to understand when we are in the middle of a trial, or if others have done us wrong. People wrong others every day. Often it is not fair, and their actions can cause us heartache and pain. Even though we have been wronged, our reaction to that person or the situation is still our choice.

We can choose to put it behind us, forgive and forget, or we can choose to carry a grudge and let it destroy our happiness. It is true that others can cause us trial or pain, but they cannot take away your happiness if we do not let them.

"People are about as happy as they make up their minds to be."

—Abraham Lincoln

Do we really believe this and live this way or is it just a nice saying? Maybe we can get through the normal trials of life, but can we really deal with the greater challenges and be positive and happy? Fortunately, many of us will never have to experience some of the terrible trials of life such as starvation, rape, or murder, but all of us have to carry our own cross, and sometimes the weight of it all might seem unbearable.

It is hard to know what to tell others in their times of trial because sometimes the weight of it all might seem too much for us to bear. But know that God has promised us relief if we place our trials on His shoulders.[285] Plus, it really does help to look at the good and be grateful for what we have in life.

When things get tough, many of us fall upon our knees and plead for God's help, as we should, but do we remember to have proper

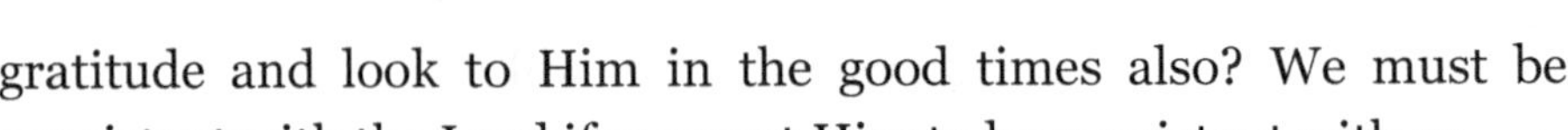

gratitude and look to Him in the good times also? We must be consistent with the Lord if we want Him to be consistent with us.

Gratitude is the best way to tune yourself into what is good to attract more of it. Through gratitude we can bring so much more into our lives. The great scientist Albert Einstein revolutionized the way we view time, space, and gravity. From his poor background and humble beginnings, you would have thought it impossible for him to achieve all that he did. Einstein had a great understanding of proper gratitude, he said, "Thank you" hundreds of times each day.[286] God is the most important being to thank; He has given us all we have, even our very lives.

Be careful to not get too discouraged when you fail at things you attempt to do, for we have all failed at something. There is no real gain without risk and with risk sometimes we fail. If you fall down again and again you are most likely learning something from it! Just make sure you get up once more than you fall down. Does God want us to continually beat ourselves up over our weaknesses and failures? It doesn't make sense He would. He just wants us to learn from them and move forward.

We will most likely treat others the way we treat ourselves, so we must be positive and loving with ourselves, and that will help us be that same way with our family and friends. Some of the greatest people in history have made many mistakes, but the mistakes were minor compared to the marvelous work they accomplished:

None of us is perfect. We all make many mistakes daily. Don't highlight your own mistakes, or those of others. Look at the greater good and be positive.

Another great way to be positive is to develop a good sense of humor. Some people just have a naturally jolly way about them, others have an amazing sense of humor, and yet others really need to loosen up and have some fun. It is fun to be around people with a

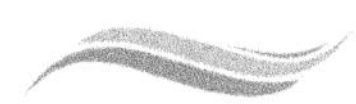

great sense of humor. We can develop these qualities. Ask God to help you laugh each day and find the humor in the ordinary.

Much of the comedy in our world is rude and crude, and often the jokes are directed toward someone else in a demeaning way. This is prideful and it may breed gossip and backbiting in others. If the comedian can make people laugh by poking fun at himself, or about life in general in a clean manner, then it's great. Red Skelton was one of the greatest of his time; the world needs more comedians like him.

Viewing some of the fun TV shows of the 60's, 70's, and 80's is a great way to escape from it all and help us take life a little less serious. Shows such as *The Munster's, Mr. Ed, Leave It to Beaver, I Dream of Jeanne, I Love Lucy, Gilligan's Island, Little House on The Prairie, Highway to Heaven, Kung Fu, Gomer Pile, Green Acres, Bewitched, The Andy Griffin Show, Hogan's Heroes, Mork and Mindy*, and *The Brady Bunch* are some of the best ever created.

There are also many great movies out that are hilarious and/ or wholesome, such as: *Enchanted, The Princess Bride, The Kid, What About Bob, Mr. Magoo, Dumb and Dumber, Bridge To Terabithia, Joan of Arc, Dreamer, Chariots of Fire, Ben Hur, The 10 Commandments, Joseph, It's a Wonderful Life, Life is Beautiful, Where The Red Fern Grows, Old Yeller, A Christmas Carol, Pride and Prejudice, Amazing Grace, Gracie, Bella, Invincible, We Are Marshall, The Pride of the Yankees, A Man For All Seasons, Miracle on 34th Street, The Ultimate Gift, The Other Side of Heaven, Night At The Museum, Tucker, October Sky, 13 Going On 30, Gone With The Wind, Father of the Bride, Simon Birch, Turner and Hooch, Miracle, Johnny Lingo, Just Like Heaven, Man From Snowy River, Akela and the Bee, Sound of Music.*

The writers and producers of these TV shows and movies deserve great respect. They bring wholesome entertainment to our world and give us opportunities to laugh and escape to a world of fantasy and fun.

The easiest way to laugh is to be around children. They laugh all the time. The average child laughs hundreds of times each day, and the average adult laughs just a few times.[287] Isn't this sad? For the adult that is. Children do really funny things. The stuff they come up with is amazing. It's like an impromptu comedy night every day. Remember to keep a light heart and not take yourself too seriously. Goethe said, "Angels fly because they take themselves lightly." Spend as much time as possible with children; re-discover the world through 4-year-old eyes.

Have an abundance mentality, not a scarcity mentality.

See abundance, feel abundance, and don't let anything or anyone convince you that there is only so much to go around. Take a look at our world, there is more than enough of everything for everyone. Some are so focused on the top, being #1, and having more than others, that they do not realize that God's plan is one of success, not failure. Billions of people that have come to this earth will get to heaven, and it doesn't matter if we get there first or last, as long as we make it. There are not only so many spots there. God doesn't grade on a curve. Each of us has a place there if through God's help we qualify. Forget about what the world teaches us about being #1. That's the way of the world, not the way of God. Forget about the guy who is ahead of you. Focus on yourself and becoming better each day.[288] Race yourself, maybe have a little competitive fun with others along the way, but don't let them mess you up. Keep your eye on the goal, *improving yourself.*

Be happy, have joy, and be positive.

"Happiness is not the absence of problems,
but the ability to deal with them."

—Steve Maraboli

You have so much talent, more than you know, and you have so much to look forward to. Our future is bright. Some doomsayers talk

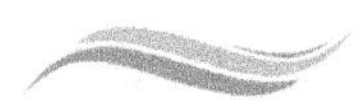

constantly about how bad everything is here in our world. Do they not believe or understand that God is in control? Don't you think if God is perfect, and if He is in control, that things will eventually turn out for the best? Of course, they will! This is one of the best reasons to stay positive and not let all the negative things in our world get us down.

It is a great thing to want more out of life than you currently have, but to base our happiness upon these things is wrong.

Again, sometimes this can be very hard in the society we live in, because so much has to do with being #1, having lots of not only the necessities of life, but also the luxuries of life, and having more of them than the person next to you. This is the world telling us what's most important. What really is most important is your relationship with God, and your relationship with your spouse and family members. If anyone or anything tries to persuade you to believe otherwise, don't be pressured into believing that way.

Let's talk more about being positive and grateful for what we have. Positive thinking has proven physiological benefits. When you think positively, the positive thoughts aren't confined to your brain. They set in motion a chain of events that has been defined physiologically. We know that expectation and suggestion achieve a lot of fabulous changes in the immune system and probably every other organ in the body. When you get into a meditative, prayer-like, contemplative frame of mind, the metabolism slows down, the immune system is refreshed, blood pressure and heart rates subside, blood lactate level falls, and oxygen consumption and carbon dioxide production are diminished. A lot of changes happen, the result of which is that the body becomes healthier. There are loads of evidence that show prayer and meditation work to make your life work better!

Look at the blessings all of us enjoy. We are alive and kicking! Most of us have families that love us. In America, we enjoy many freedoms and liberties that other people throughout the world only dream of. Most of us have many of not only the necessities of life,

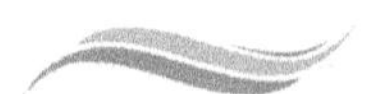

but also many of the luxuries of life. Many of us are in the top 99.999 percentile in the world in what we have. We have education available to us through school and literature. We have many choices for our careers, the opportunity to raise healthy, educated children, the blessing to worship God as we choose, our homes, cars, and comforts in life. We have opportunities to travel, serve others, feel love, and see the beauties of the earth. We have unlimited capacities, amazing mental abilities, our physical bodies, and a host of other blessings if we just consider them for a moment. Even breath itself is a privilege. All these things are given to us from God for our enjoyment and benefit.

It is interesting to be around older people. Just an observation; it seems like they are more on the extremes than younger people. It seems like they have either learned through life's experiences to enjoy life and look at the positive, being grateful for what they've been given, or it seems like they have not learned, and are bitter and ungrateful. Many do not appreciate life and all the opportunities it affords them. Many times, we forget how blessed we are. We complain and wallow in our own problems. We are so fortunate to have a loving Heavenly Father who will forgive us of our weaknesses and shortcomings. How truly blessed we are.

QUESTION EVERYTHING?
DAD,
WERE DID GOD
COME FROM?
QETommy.com

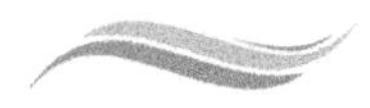

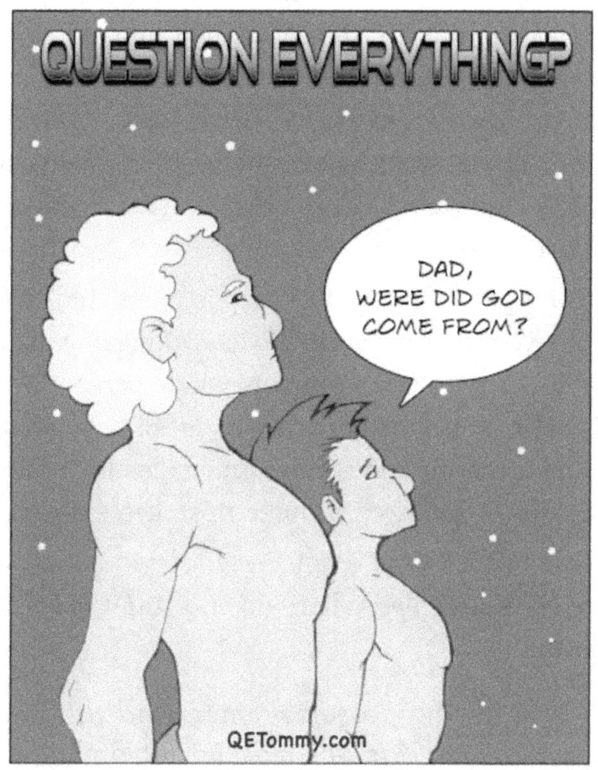

PRINCIPLE #2 – Rely Upon God

You cannot do it alone

Many of the greatest minds to ever live have said it; we must rely upon a power greater than ourselves.[289] We cannot do it all alone, no matter how motivated, focused, disciplined, our strong we are. Sooner or later, we must bring God, or a Higher Power, into the equation, or we will end up a lost soul.[290] People might end up with what they want in life, but it often isn't what is most important, or what will make them happy. The world is full of people who have achieved much success in life but are miserable. How can this be if they are able to achieve what they set out to do and are living their dreams? It is because they are out of balance, BodyMindSpirit. We are only as strong as our weakest link. If our focus has been to achieve success in one area, but we have disregarded other areas, we will never be happy or fulfilled. Yes, it will feel great at the top, but reality will soon set in, and we know who we really are. We can never escape the truth no matter how hard we try.

Does this mean everyone at the top is miserable? Of course not. Many who achieve their dreams in life have done it while maintaining the balance necessary to be a complete whole person, and have done it with God's help. Nothing is drastically out of balance. If they make mistakes, which everyone does, these mistakes are often just errors in judgment. They often do not make mistakes knowingly; they are living up to what they know to be true.

How is your character? Where do you stand in life? Are you on the side of truth?

"I hope I shall always possess firmness and virtue enough to maintain what I consider the most enviable of all titles, the character of an honest man."

—George Washington

Alcoholics Anonymous, one of the most successful programs for personal change in America's history, is centered on the principle that in order to change, and have it be permanent, we must rely upon a power greater than ourselves. Would they have the great success they have achieved if they left this true principle out? No. There might not even be such a program if they left God out of the equation. How can we accomplish our greatest desires in life without God? We can't.

"When the Great Scorer comes to write against your name, He marks, not that you won or lost, but how you played the game."

—Grantland Rice

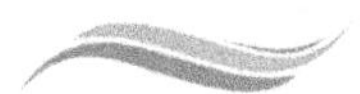

How are you playing the game? If we let God into our life. He will make more of us than we could ever imagine.

QUESTION EVERYTHING?
MOM, DO FIREWORKS MEAN SOMEONE IS KISSING?
QETommy.com

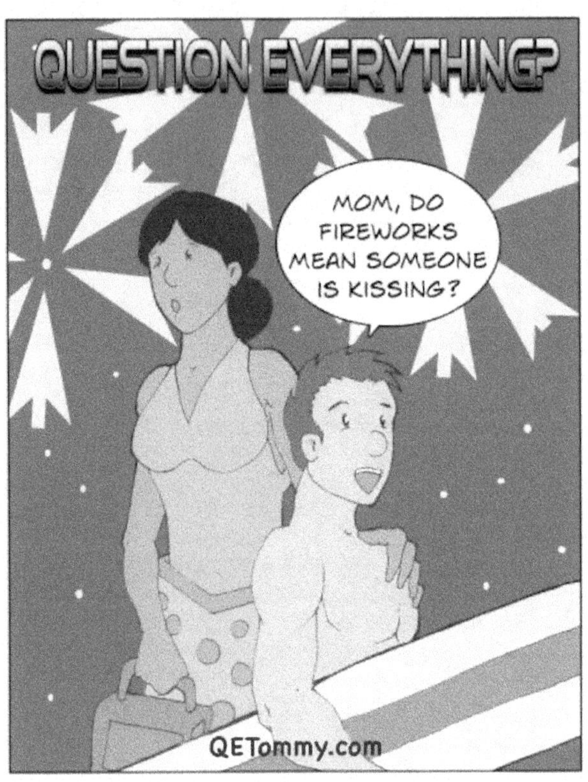

PRINCIPLE # 3 – Dream

And make your dream reality everyday

Dreeeeaaam dream dream...there's a song about that. Whatever you can dream go do it. It's been said whatever you can conceive and believe you can achieve. Be an active dreamer, not a passive one, by making your dreams reality every day.

This should be one of our favorite things to do in life, because everything begins with our thoughts, and we are free to think whatever we desire.

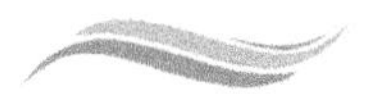

"Man's mind, once stretched by a new idea, never regains its original dimension."

Oliver Wendell Holmes

Active dreaming should be exciting. If this process is not exciting to you, you are doing something wrong. It was Einstein who told us that imagination is more important than knowledge. Create your future by imagining it first. Don't just wander through life being a product of your environment, circumstances, or lot in life. Even if you are born in the best possible circumstances imaginable, make things better for you, your family, and your posterity. Nobody is perfect, there is always room for improvement.

"Some goals are so worthy, it's glorious even to fail."

—Captain Manoj Kumar Pandey

Maybe you want to play baseball in the Major Leagues. Yes, one out of a million kids actually get to do it, but why not you? Go make a million dollars. Marry a chorus girl. Be happy. Develop the talents you've been blessed with. Sing in front of 10,000 people. Raise the best kids you've ever known. Develop the kind of personality that people love. Be fulfilled. Have true joy. Buy that car. Live in that house. Have your own company. Never raise your voice to your spouse (unless there's a fire). Speak kindly to your kids. Get that raise. Work less than 40 hours a week. Golf three times a week. Get your body fat under 15%. Have a happy marriage. Have more energy. Sleep eight hours a night. Get straight A's. Take that vacation. Move to Hawaii. Bike across America. Have good friends. Learn how to defend yourself. Win that race. Be top 10 in your age group. Make the Olympic Team. Read all those volumes. Hire that coach. Go talk to that person. Get off the Prozac. Get the love and romance back. Find your soul mate. You can do it. But it must first begin with your thoughts and dreams in your mind. Thoughts become real things. This is how God created the world; this is how your perfect life must be created.

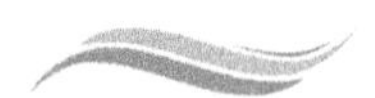

Begin by writing down everything you want to accomplish in your lifetime, preferably in a journal, so you don't lose it and can refer to it from time to time. Again, this should not be a chore, rather something that is fun and exciting. If it's a chore, you are doing something wrong. Get excited about your life. Get out of that rut or hole you are in. Take life by the horns and be all that you can be. But first, you need to think it up. Anything you really believe you can do in life, and want to do, write it down. You might be amazed as you look back at this list in a few years from now. If you are on course your life will come together, and some of these things you hoped for but didn't know for sure you could achieve, you will achieve. You can live your dreams.

Things might not go as planned, and sometimes we need to be very patient, but God places desires in our hearts, ones that really are possible, and if we are faithful to these dreams God will provide a way for them to be fulfilled.[291] So, get that journal out and have at it. Maybe write 100-200 goals down, or just start writing and then stop when you are done. It might take you awhile, or everything might just flow quickly. Break your goals up into 4 sections, Fitness, Nutrition, Mind, and Spirit. This is Key; you don't want 100 goals under fitness but only 5 goals under mind. Granted, some goals are going to be bigger than others, and will take much more energy and determination to achieve. So, you likely won't have the same number in each section, just be conscious of balance and synergy between these four sections. If you have a hard time thinking of goals in a particular section, maybe use this book, or others related to your body, mind, or spirit, to help you come up with goals in each section. Remember, this process should be exciting to you. Don't make it so labor intensive that it is not fun.

Here's an example of 4-7 goals in each of four sections: Fitness, Nutrition, Mind & Spirit:

Fitness

1. Stay regularly involved (twice per week) in a sport
2. Keep my body fat under 20%

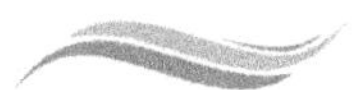

3. Exercise at least 4 times per week
4. Squats at least once per week

Nutrition

1. Eat 70% whole foods
2. Have great energy
3. Never use medication long term
4. No food after 8pm

Mind

1. Read 1 new book per month
2. Have a clean and organized home
3. Listen to good music everyday
4. Write in my journal every day
5. Work less than 40 hours a week
6. Make new monthly goals on the 1st of each month
7. Have a collection of great wholesome movies for the family

Spirit

1. Date with wife once a week
2. Spend time with each child each day
3. Go to Church every week
4. Pray at least twice a day
5. Read the scriptures everyday
6. Pray for control of anger
7. Say thanks at least 10 times a day

"Well done is better than well said."

—Benjamin Franklin

How exactly do we make our dreams or goals reality? You must *work* on your dreams every day, or they will never be anything more than this, a dream. Will you make the Major Leagues if you never practice? It will never happen. It doesn't matter how much talent you've been blessed with. You might need to practice more than anyone else because you might not have as much natural talent as most other Major Leaguers. But if you had to put in twice as much work as anyone else to get there, and you still get there, nobody will ever be able to take this away from you. When you are out on the field playing with that guy who put in less work than you, does anyone care? All anyone really cares about is what you do that day, and if you are better, you win. If you lose, you still win. Because you did so much more just to be there.

"Anything is possible with ordinary talent and extraordinary perseverance."

—Thomas Fowell Buxton

Maybe your Major League in life is having your own successful company, raising great kids, or securing your life financially. Whatever it is, do it every day, make it happen with God's help, and you will be truly happy, satisfied, and fulfilled. What greater things can we do in life?

QUESTION EVERYTHING?
DAD,
HOW COME THAT GUY
DIDN'T WASH HIS
HANDS AFTER GOING
#2?
RESTROOMS
MEN
QETommy.com

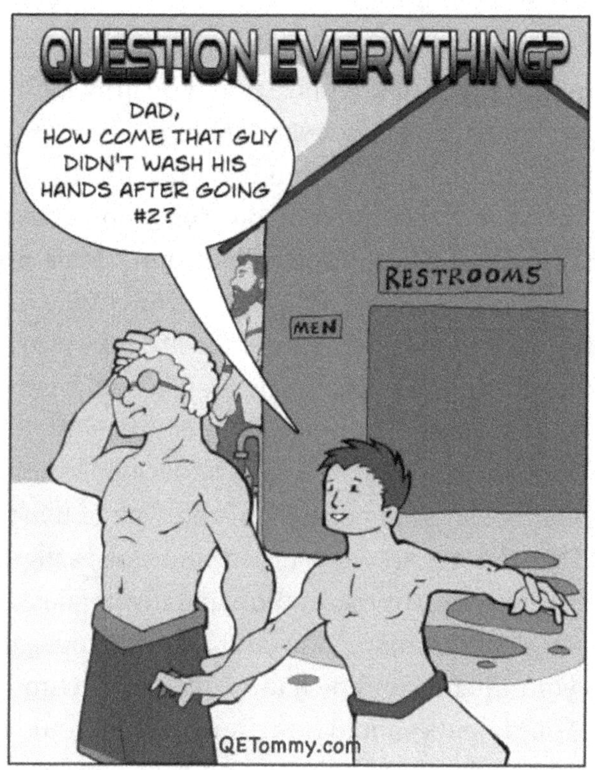

PRINCIPLE #4
Organize Your Life
Create a Proactive Mind

"If I had six hours to chop down a tree, I'd spend the first four hours sharpening the saw."

—Abraham Lincoln

This is what you're doing by dreaming, setting goals, writing them down, preparing a mission statement, reading this book...you

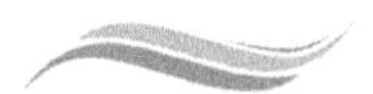

are sharpening your saw. You are very wise. It will make the actual labor so much easier and enjoyable.

What are your greatest talents? It's not healthy for us to compare our talents to others to make us feel better than others, but it's healthy to compare to figure out just what our specific talents are so we can develop them. "Compete with your old self." Sometimes this takes much thought and reflection, especially if our talents are those that are hard to compare to others. It's easy to run a race and figure out if we came in first or last, although we need to take into account how much training and effort went into our preparation, versus how much those around us have put in to make a fair assessment. But it's harder to figure out things such as strengths and weakness for a particular career, personality traits we possess, or the type of marriage partner that's best. The options are very broad and not easily quantifiable. This is where prayer and/or meditation and deep reflection comes in. God knows you better than anyone, and He will guide you to discern and develop your talents, and be happy, if you ask Him to do so. The developing of our talents should be a major focus in our lives, because it is one that will bring us much joy and satisfaction. Everyone has talent within but most don't have the courage to let their talent lead them to their greatest destiny.

We need to pattern our lives after correct principles of the universe or the principles of happiness. If you do not have any idea what these principles are, do some searching. Read good books, talk to people who you think are truly happy and satisfied, and learn the lessons of history. Look at others who are happy people. Often, they are not the ones in the spotlight, so you might need to do some digging. Look to your ancestors. Read their journals if they had them. Learn about them and what they went through in their lives. Take the good and throw out the bad and apply their best examples to your life. It might amaze you how in tune you really are with the principles of

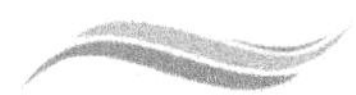

happiness. There is no other way to be happy, have true joy, and be at peace than to follow these principles.

Get in tune with your purpose here on earth and don't waste time. Time is precious.

"Don't confuse activity with accomplishment!"

—Zig Ziggler

Spend your time on things that matter most, things that will help you accomplish your desired results.

Watching sleazy TV shows and movies is an example of what *not* to do in our spare time. How much time last week did you spend watching TV that has no lasting value? If you said zero, you are to be congratulated. Yes, there are many shows on TV that are very valuable and not at all a waste of time. Yes, entertainment is an important part of life, sometimes we just need to relax and not do much of anything at all, maybe watch something funny that makes us laugh, or is thought provoking and entertaining. But when the average household in America has the TV on 4-6 hours a day something is drastically wrong. Why do people watch so much TV? Maybe it is because their own lives are so boring? Maybe they are looking for an escape into a fantasy world? Or maybe it's because they have no great goals in life, or are discouraged? Many have jobs where they do not feel any great challenge, enjoyment, or excitement, so they just go through the motions figuring this is about as good as life gets and they do whatever it takes to just hang in there. TV, alcohol, or drugs are all forms of escape from reality. Sure, life can be really hard at times, and there are many times when we just need to hang in there until things get better, but if this is a constant in our life, we need to make some changes.

Why do so many settles for lives of mediocrity? Why would anyone in their right mind choose to not live a happy, fulfilling life?

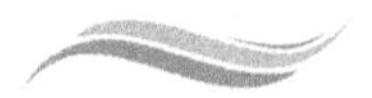

Fear is a big one. Fear is the opposite of faith. How do we get over it? Exhibit some courage.

"Courage is resistance to fear, mastery of fear, not absence of fear."

—Mark Twain

Most of us are afraid of someone or something. We must conquer that fear and exercise faith and courage.

"What matters is not the size of the dog in the fight, but the size of the fight in the dog"

—Coach Bear Bryant

Many escape depression by just staying busy, and there is much to be said for just getting out and doing something. But why are we doing what we're doing? The most successful people in life always have a purpose for most everything they do. Read about them. Al Oerter, a 4-time Olympic Gold Medal discus thrower, says he thought about it (winning a gold medal) almost all day long every day; when he ate, when he went to bed at night, when he was working out, when he was resting, when he was showering. His mind was constantly focused on the task at hand.[292] There were others who were maybe more talented, and others did have more world records, but it was Al who always came up with the gold medal in the Olympic Games. Some might say he just got lucky, or it just happened to be his day on Olympic Day. Others who know better understand that Al willed it to happen through his thought process and hard work.

Jerry Rice, now there's a guy who is an inspiration. Do you think Jerry spent most of his time in football working on things that are urgent and not important? Not a chance. How about Benjamin Franklin, Alexander Graham Bell, Abe Lincoln, and Philo T. Farnsworth? These people failed so many times it's just amazing to read their life stories. What force kept them going? They were driven to succeed by their

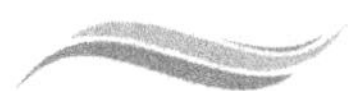

focus, hard work, mental imagery, and living in accordance with the principles of success. They paid the price and were rewarded for their efforts. The same holds true for us. If we are driven by a cause greater than ourselves, even if we are not in perfect harmony with correct principles of the Universe, we can still accomplish our objectives. We don't need to be perfect. Only one person has ever done that, Christ Himself, but we do need to be within the realm of possibility. Whether your goal might be to raise great kids and/or become a Major Leaguer, *you can do it.*

Let's talk briefly about cleanliness and having orderly surroundings.

"Sometimes when I consider what tremendous consequences come from the little things, I am tempted to think... there are no little things."

—Bruce Barton

Being neat and clean might seem like such a little thing to so many people, a thing that takes time away from doing what we really want to do or need to do. The necessities of life are important. Our life revolves around work, whether it's mental, physical, or spiritual labor. We must always be engaged in a good cause and do many things of our own free will.[293] This includes being neat and clean.

Cleanliness is next to Godliness.[294] Can you imagine going to heaven when you die and it being a mess? Organize your life, put first things first; get your physical environment under control, so you have the ability to organize the rest of your life. You have responsibilities here on earth. Don't shirk them. Take them to heart and do the best you can with them.

We live in a society that doesn't place as much emphasis on the importance of motherhood as we should. Many men do not understand the work and labor that it takes to run a household and raise children. These men need to take a "vacation" and come try it

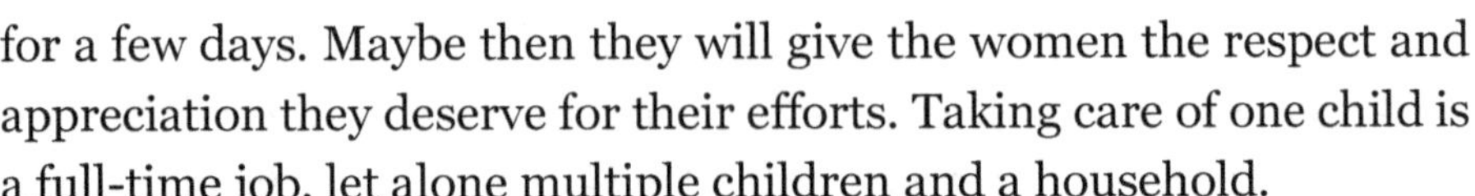

for a few days. Maybe then they will give the women the respect and appreciation they deserve for their efforts. Taking care of one child is a full-time job, let alone multiple children and a household.

"I am distressed that the modern world's devaluation of motherhood is signaling to my daughter and her friends that preparing to be a homemaker, mother, and wife is 'no big deal'...In truth, learning to be a superb mother is a very big deal...Such a task involves creating and maintaining a total environment of human warmth, intellectual stimulation, and spiritual strength by someone who sees the wellsprings of personal meaning that lie beyond a first glance at a diaper, a frying pan, and a worn tennis shoe."

—Marie K. Hafen

The importance of motherhood will be discussed in more length in the principles of a healthy spirit, but may it be said here that this includes both the husband and wife.

"Your success as a family – our success as a society – depends not on what happens at the White House, but what happens inside your house."

—Barbara Bush

Part of this work at home includes creating a neat and clean environment for our families.

Some women try to be Superwomen and do it all--raise kids, work, clean, cook, community service...*slow down!* God does *not* expect us to run faster than we are able.[295] Delegate more, have your husband and children help out. Tell them you cannot do it all. Don't do it all. Take time for yourself, or you will get burnt out and will not succeed at what's most important, being a good wife and mother. Husbands, pick up the slack. Don't expect her to do everything, spread out the work between you. Help around the house, be of good cheer, make the work fun. Don't sit in front of the TV while she's up working. She

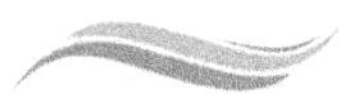

was at it all day just like you. If she cooks, you do the dishes, or maybe do everything together.

Work together, then sit down together and relax together. Enjoy each other's company. Be a partner and a best friend. Maybe you need to figure out how to make more money at your work so your wife does not have to work? This does not necessarily mean more work for you, just work *smarter*. Or maybe just be happy without that boat or new car. What's more important, that boat, or your wife at home when the children come home from school? Pray to God for help, and He will inspire you to be a better provider, husband, and father.

Teach your children to work, first by setting a good example, then by teaching them to be self-sufficient. Do not pick up after them if they are capable of doing it themselves. It might take more time to teach them when they are young, but in the long run your house will be a lot cleaner, and you will not be doing all the work. "*Whatever you take out put back*", and *"Clean up after yourself"* are good family sayings. Maybe put them up somewhere in the house so everyone remembers them. By teaching children to be neat and clean, you will create an atmosphere of learning and growth. Their future spouses will thank you, and life will be much easier if everyone is cooperating and helping out, working toward the common good. Good hygiene will help your children be successful in their social interactions and help them to find a person that also values good hygiene and cleanliness. Like attracts like. If you want them to marry someone who is neat and clean, then teach them to be this way. Your time and energy will be worth every effort.

"When an old person dies, a library is lost."

—Tommy Swanson

Will this be true of you? Or will we lose a mind filled with cheap entertainment and useless information? It is said that the majority of college graduates will never again in their lifetime read a book cover

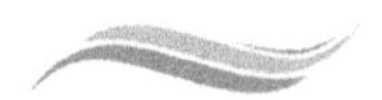

to cover.[296] How could this be? If this is true it is a sad state of affairs. A story in the *New York Times* published a study entitled; "Study Says Half of Adults in U.S. Lack Reading and Math Abilities", offered some sobering statistics based on a study of more than 26,000 Americans above age fifteen.

> Nearly half of the nation's 191 million adult citizens are not proficient enough in English to write a letter about a billing error or to calculate the length of a bus trip from a published schedule, according to a four-year Federal study. The study, released yesterday by the Education Department, presented a bleak statistical portrait of the nation's literacy...Businesses estimate they lose $25 billion to $30 billion a year nationwide in lost productivity, errors and accidents attributed to poor literacy.

We live in an age where people want to be entertained constantly. The average household has the TV on about 4-5 hours a day. The average father talks to his child 7 minutes per day, and the average mother talks to her child 11 minutes per day.[297] Are you average? How can we create a happy, healthy, productive life when we spend so much time being entertained, and so little time with those we love? What are we doing to ourselves, and our families? Who's really raising our children? When we see a movie, watch TV, or see a video where the entertainment industry does all the creative work for us, where we just sit back, relax, and let the movie create an escape to a world of fantasy, we are not using our own marvelous minds. There is nothing wrong with a good movie or TV show, or a relaxing evening of not doing much of anything, but to never read a book cover to cover after college, and to talk to our children only 7-11 minutes a day?

"Those who do not read good books have no advantage over those who cannot read them."

—Mark Twain

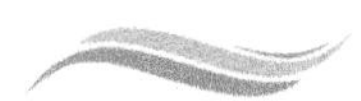

How educated are we really? That college degree makes you more valuable in your workplace, but does it make you a more valuable individual? If we are so much the products of our environments, what kind of environment are you creating for you, your spouse, and/or children? Is it any wonder there are so many depressed, lonely, and discouraged people? Are we surprised so many people watch so much TV, take illegal drugs, get drunk, take anti-depressants, and generally live lives of mediocrity, never living up to their true potential and be all that they can be?

"Television is perhaps the greatest medium ever discovered to teach and educate and even to entertain. But the filth, the rot, the violence, and the profanity that spew from the television screens into our homes is deplorable. It is a sad commentary on our society. The fact that a television is on six or seven hours a day in most of the homes of America says something of tremendous importance. A study by the American Psychological Association determined that a typical child who begins, at the age of three years, to watch twenty-seven hours of TV a week, will view 8,000 murders and 100,000 acts of violence by the age of twelve years... It is naïve to believe that a steady diet of blatant immorality, played out nightly in our living rooms, has no effect on people. I am always curious when individuals insist that what they watch on television or in a movie theatre doesn't affect them. It was interesting to note that the going rate for a thirty-second advertising spot for the 1999 Super Bowl was 1.5 million dollars. Apparently, a host of advertisers felt confident that in 30 seconds' time they could influence their viewers to buy the products or services they were peddling. Are we really to believe that hours, leading to years, of television viewing will not affect attitudes about everything from family life to appropriate sexual relations?"

—Gordon B. Hinckley

Each year the average child watches approximately 22,000 commercials; 5,000 of them for food products, the majority of which

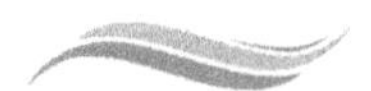

are high-calorie, high-sugar, low-nutrition items. Research indicates that 67 percent of Saturday morning commercials are for sugared cereals, candy bars, and other sweets. Only 3 percent of TV food ads are for fruits and vegetables.[298] Clearly, television does not promote healthy nutrition.

There's nothing wrong with being entertained a few hours each week. In fact, it is probably healthy. But when it consumes our spare time, maybe we need to make some changes? Take charge of your life and create a proactive mind. Reading good books allows your mind to create those mental images, instead of being fed them on a silver platter, and often the silver screen hollows in comparison (even with their millions of dollars and the latest and greatest visual effects) to a really creative mind. Great minds will be curious.

If we are curious, we will want to know what is in the classics, we will want to know about the world we live in, we will be interested in people and in other cultures.

Keeping a journal is another great way to create a great mind. In a good acting school this is one of the first things they will have you do, keep a journal.[299] Why? Because it helps us get more in tune with ourselves, and to be more creative. These are very valuable acting skills that also transfer over to our daily lives. If you are diligent in your journal keeping, not only will you gain a better command of your native language and develop very useful communication skills, which will obviously help you in school or in the workplace, you will also have time to think out loud and create your perfect world. These things are invaluable if you really want to be all that you can be because everything begins with what we think about.

Who do you think will have an easier time picturing their perfect world in their minds and creating it, the person who watches countless hours of entertainment on TV or Internet, or the person who reads great books, keeps a journal, and has learned to create those mental images themselves? Everything begins with what we think about. We

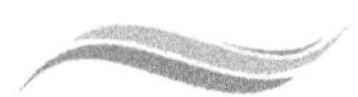

create our own destinies. If our minds are creative and sharp, our lives will reflect this training. We will more likely achieve what we want in life, and be happy and fulfilled, not products of our environments, but masters of our own souls, and creators of our own destinies.

Many know how to create a healthy body through proper nutrition and exercise, even though many times they do not do it, they nevertheless know what needs to be done. But many do not apply this same logic to the mind. They cannot understand why they are depressed, lonely, or mentally weak. It is hard for them to comprehend why they give in so easy to alcohol abuse, drugs, adultery, violence, or the other corrupting influences that surround us. Their minds are weak because they have not used them, or focused them, on the right things. At 80 years of age will your mind be as sharp (or sharper) then it is today? The choice is yours.

These thoughts are not new. They are the basics of life, and they are built on truth and logic. It is so easy to overlook the basics, get caught up in the world, and never achieve our true potential and be truly happy. It's so sad.

"What is the mystery...about a society that has the manners of a rock band, the morals of a soap opera, the decision-making ability of the Simpson's and wants to pay for Government with Visa or American Express? Why should we be surprised that our underlying culture is constructed from the ratings-based, give-them-what-they-want remote-controlled, quick-zap world of commercial television?"

—Former Editor - *Chicago Tribune*

The purpose here is not to bash TV or the Internet. These are some of the greatest inventions ever created. But as with most things, they can be a powerful force for good or evil, depending on their use. There are so many good programs on TV, and uplifting information on the Internet, both those that are purely entertaining, and those that are educational. Watch these. But it is getting increasingly difficult to find good entertainment that is not latent with foul language, sexual innuendos, and violence; if we are what we think about, these things will affect us, no matter how short the scene or how mild the language and acts. The mind is an amazing thing; it can recall whatever it has viewed over decades of time. Unlike drugs or alcohol that will be out of our system in time, our minds never forget. This is why pornography is so destructive. It produces scenes that are sacred and should only be in a marriage relationship and allows these images to be viewed by someone other than a spouse. If these images cloud your mind, can you ever be truly faithful to one person? Not just physical faithfulness, it is more than that, can you give your whole self to your spouse, BodyMindSpirit, or just parts? Will you be with your spouse but be thinking of someone else? If so, are you really giving your whole self to that person? You can't fake it. People who are really in tune with themselves and others know what's going on.

Now, we have all made many mistakes in life, and where there have been mistakes there is forgiveness and hope...but be careful. We are playing with fire if we take these negative influences into our life.

Why do so many people live in the glory days? If we are always living in the past, what does that say about the present? Shouldn't we each have our best year in life this year? Even if life is hard for you right now...

"People are generally as happy as they make up their minds to be."

—Abe Lincoln

This same logic applies to the books we read and the things we write about. There is a lot of sleaze in our world, and garbage out there on the bookshelves. If you learn to develop a really creative mind by reading and writing, and you read and write the bad stuff, it might be even worse than viewing them on TV, or on the computer screen. What is the good stuff? Anything that is uplifting, things that encourage you to be your best self. In your journal talk about your dreams and desires in life, what you really want to accomplish. How

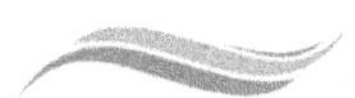

are you going to get there? Are you seeking God's help with your desires? Write down your spiritual experiences each day and mention the things you did for other people. Focus on the good things that happened to you each day. Maybe mention some of the bad, but don't dwell on them. Remember, most likely your children, grandchildren, great-grandchildren...will read your journals one day, so try to set a good example for them and be your best self.

As for reading, the Bible is the best place to start. Religious authors like C. S. Lewis are wonderful. Relationship and organizational behavioral authors like Dale Carnegie, Stephen Covey, Og Mandino, Norman Vincent Peale, Napoleon Hill, Jack Canfield and Mark Victor Hansen will change your life. Then there are the classic novels; authors like Victor Hugo creating things like *Les Misérables*, and *The Hunchback of Notre Dame*...you will never be bored with authors and books like these in your hands and minds. Read these authors and all the other books you can find that are wholesome and uplifting.

Search out things you are interested in, things that will help you accomplish your objectives in life. Keep a journal that is a treasure of your life experiences full of learning and truth, both for you and your posterity. If you do some of these things, you will soon find a peace and joy enter your life that you might not have ever known.

Now that you have some of your dreams or goals in life written down (Principle #3), or are at least thinking about doing it, let's talk about taking things a step further. Some of your goals might be lifetime goals, others might be yearly goals, and others might be monthly or weekly goals. Organize them into lifetime, 5-year, and 1-year goals in each of the 3 sections, Body, Mind & Spirit. If you really want to get specific, you can break them up further into monthly and weekly goals. Maybe set new yearly goals at the beginning of each new year, so you can see how you did during the last year and plan for the next.

Your vacation time around Christmas or New Year's would be a great time to do it. This is how to plan your life. Do it with prayer and even fasting, because God knows you a whole lot better than you do, and He will inspire you in this process. He loves you perfectly and He wants all the best things for you. He wants you to be all that you can be, and He wants you to be happy. If you are in tune with Him, He will not lead you astray.

Here's an example with 3 goals in each 4 sections: Fitness, Nutrition, Mind & Spirit

Fitness – Lifetime

1. Be physically strong and look good in the mirror
2. Be able to play any sport with my grandkids
3. No lasting injuries

Fitness – 5 years

1. Dead lift 400 pounds
2. Play two different sports competitively each year
3. Stay within striking distance of best performances

Fitness – 1-year

1. Dead lift 350 pounds
2. Play in competitive basketball league
3. Stretch everyday

Fitness – 1 month

1. Dead lift twice per week
2. Find a 30+ age baseball team to play with
3. Strengthen stomach daily

Nutrition – Lifetime

1. Eat healthy and be a good example to others
2. Live a long and vital life
3. Look good in the mirror

Nutrition – 5-Years

1. Keep body fat under 15%
2. Focus nutrition on whole grains, legumes, fruits & veggies
3. Fresh squeezed or blended juice daily

Nutrition – 1-Year

1. Read 5 good books on nutrition
2. Little or no processed foods
3. Eat at least 5 different fruits and vegetables a day

Nutrition – 1-Month

1. Buy a new juicer
2. Start a garden
3. Eat at least 70% whole foods

Mind - Lifetime

1. Be happy and find true joy in life with my wife
2. Create our perfect life together as a family
3. Focus on the good and uplifting not the corrupting influences

Mind - 5 year

1. Buy $50,000 worth of gold and silver
2. Get a collection of 100 inspiring movies
3. Retire by age 50 working less than 40 hours per week

Mind - 1 year

1. Have a 2 year supply of food
2. Read 12 good books this year
3. Pay off the car loan

Mind - 1 month

1. Get the shed cleaned and organized
2. Write in my journal 5+ times per week
3. Delegate more at work so I go home by 5pm

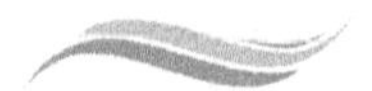

Spirit – Lifetime

1. Have a wonderful and happy marriage
2. Raise great kids
3. Have a close relationship with God

Spirit – 5-Years

1. Have a fun/ romantic date night each week with spouse
2. Help kids discover and develop their interests and talents
3. Feel closer to God each year

Spirit – 1-Year

1. Make sure I attend Church every week
2. Get each child involved in 2 different activities
3. Read the Old Testament start to finish

Spirit – 1-Month

1. Take spouse to Phantom of the Opera
2. Have a weekly date with each child
3. Read through Leviticus

Now that have you written *your* goals out, let's create your Personal Mission Statement. Your Personal Mission Statement will be something you can look at in times of trial, when you are tempted to get off course or need encouragement, something that will keep you on track to your designed destination. Something you hang on your wall, or have on your desk at work, it will be a constant reminder of your great goals and aspirations in life.

"When you were born, you cried, and the world rejoiced.
Live your life in such a manner that when you die
the world cries, and you rejoice."

—Old Indian Saying

Plot your course so the world cries at your passing. Create a

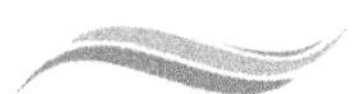

roadmap. Excellence is NEVER an accident. Sometimes this can be very hard to create because it's hard many times to see much beyond about five years into our future, but we can write down some basics that can guide us throughout our lives, and then through meditation and discernment, and/or prayer and fasting, we can chart a course that will take us where we want to go.

The first step is to begin with the end in mind. Where do you want to end up? What do you want said about you at your funeral? What will your family and friends say about you when you die, or when you see them after this life? Will they say, he (or she) was a very giving person, had many friends, worked hard, and helped many others along the way?

There is a story told about a man named J. Golden Kimball.[300] He was a respected church leader and was getting on in years. He said people would come to him all the time asking really goofy questions about the afterlife; he supposed because they knew he would be going there soon. Well, one day this lady came to him and explained that she had two brothers. One was a saint; he worked hard, was true to his wife, helped others in the community, didn't drink or smoke, everybody loved him. Then she had another brother who was bad news. He was drunk all the time, cheated on his wife, did whatever he could to get ahead, and was generally disliked by most everyone. Now the lady said, "My good brother died last fall, leaving behind a beautiful wife and family, and my other brother is still alive being as mean and rowdy as ever. Where's the justice in that?" J. Golden looked at the lady and said, "Well, I guess the good Lord doesn't want that worthless brother of yours around anymore than you do!" ☺ Figure out what you want others to say about you when your life is over; this is a great place to start.

Once you have organized your thoughts and written down some of your great goals in life, create your Personal Mission Statement, which will be your personal roadmap to success. How do you create it? Just start writing, don't worry if everything isn't perfect. You can fine-tune it later. How long should it be? That's up to you. A general guideline might be 1-3 paragraphs in length. When you are done, stop. If you think there needs to be more added, keep going. Although it's a very personal experience, here's an example of a Personal Mission Statement to give you a model upon which to create your own. This process might take you several weeks, or you might be able to do it in a day. It really depends on how much thought you've put into all this before you sit down to write. You can always add to it through the years. Nothing is set in stone, as you grow and progress in life you should gain greater perspective and understanding of what you were sent here to do, your special purpose in life

Personal Mission Statement

I will love the Lord and do what He wants me to do. I will be an influence for good because of my love for others, the talents I have developed, and for the faith I possess. I will acknowledge His blessings in my life so I carry a grateful heart and give credit where it is due, to Him.

Other than my relationship with the Lord, my wife will be my greatest concern. I will love and care for her most tenderly. Together we will be a dynamic team. Our children will be loved, cherished, and treated fairly. They will be brought up in the ways of the Lord and know we have prayed with much faith concerning them. Our home will be a place of comfort, enjoyment, and peace to all who enter. In my workplace I will excel and always strive to better myself. I will get much satisfaction out of my work because of my talent, hard work, honesty, and vision. In my community and church service, I will magnify whatever I'm asked to do and not care about the title or position, but only care about those I serve. I will have many friends and those relationships will be deep and meaningful. I will be a scholar of the best books and be more than learned – I will possess

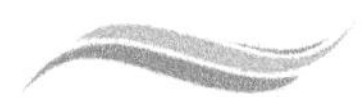

wisdom and knowledge. My life will be full of light and love and joy because I'm true to the principles that govern them.

Hopefully this will help you as you create a mission statement that will be your personal roadmap to happiness and success in your life.

Once you have established these dreams, goals, and desires, stick to them; especially if you have fasted and prayed about them, and feel good about them.

Some may try to discourage you, even those close to you, but stay focused.

"Keep away from people who try to belittle your ambitions. Small people always do that, but the really great make you feel that you, too, can become great."

—Mark Twain

Focus each day on these dreams and goals and work hard each day on the most important tasks at hand in their accomplishment.

QUESTION EVERYTHING?
HEY DAD,
IF ELECTRIC CARS GET LIKE
250 MILES/ GALLON, WHY
DON'T WE ALL DRIVE THEM?
QETommy.com

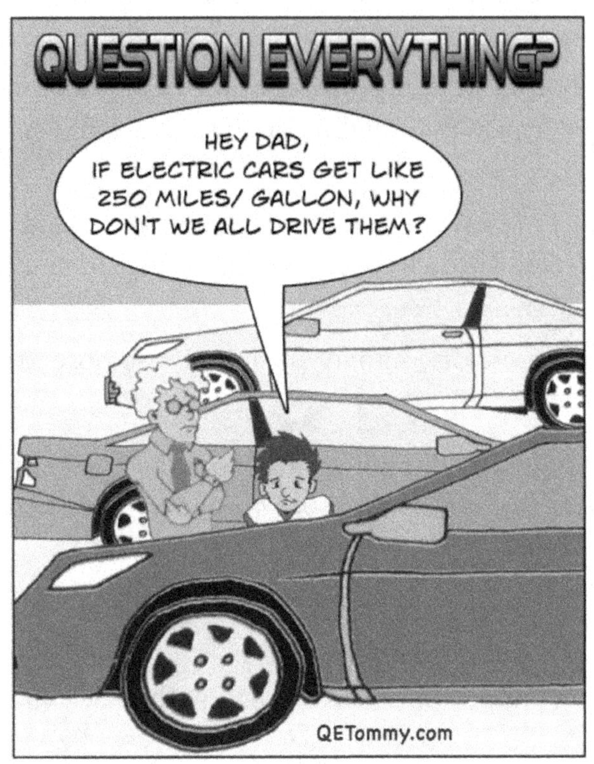

PRINCIPLE #5
Become Financially Secure
Set Yourself Free

You are the one who needs to take charge of your financial future. You are responsible for your financial security and making sure you are wise with your money. Just like in the rest of their lives, most people just go with the flow and react to their financial future, rather than accepting responsibility and taking charge (acting). Eight out of ten people polled do not have a written financial plan.[301] Why? Maybe because it seems easier, and it is what most of their friends

and parents have done. Why should they do anything different? They will most likely get nowhere financially unless they get lucky and just fall into something good, and where will they end up? According to a Social Security Administration report, nine out of ten people (90%) at 65 years of age are either dead or dead broke.[302] Because of laziness, fear, and ignorance most will not do much of anything to secure their financial futures and blow any extra money they may have on things that don't get anyone anywhere...what a waste. Be wise, get informed, and go do something good with the money you earn; *earn interest, don't pay it.*[303]

This can be tough in today's world. Not because it's so hard to do, but because we are so driven by advertising, keeping up with the Jones's, and living on the edge...we end up being far from wise. But it is possible to be wise and prudent with our money, if we follow some basic principles of good money management.

Today more than 2.8 billion people live in poverty, which is about 50% of the world's population. This poverty is defined as having an income of less than $2 a day.[304] We have more poor people than at any other time in our history.

Although the percentage of poor people in the world's total population is actually improving, because of the wealth-creating power of industrial development, the gap between the rich and poor is rising.[305]

There has never been more of a separation between the rich and the poor as there is today, and this separation will likely only continue to expand. The world is getting increasingly wicked, and the rich will not share with the poor. Many of the rich figure they are smarter, work harder, and thus deserve what they have. This is not true, poor people many times are smarter and work much harder than the rich.

The best way to overcome the financial hardships that afflict the poor is through education, both a financial education, and a college

education.[306] It is a proven fact that people who have a college degree make substantially more money than those who do not, and those who have a Master's Degree earn more than those who just have a Bachelor's Degree, and so on up the list.[307] So the safest and most secure way to ensure your financial future is through education. This is not to say if you do not have a college degree, or do not have any desire to get one, that you will never be financially secure. It just makes things more difficult. So, the first suggestion for financial security in your life, and in your family's life, is to go to school, as much as possible. Set aside college funds for your children as soon as they are born so they can go to school too.

Now, let's talk about your *financial education*. This is the most important factor in becoming financially free and living the good life financially.[308] Most times our educational system teaches people how to work for other people. As Wyatt Earp said long ago, "You will never get rich working for someone else." Don't quit your job in haste and start your own business, though this might be the best thing you could ever do. Simply take charge of your financial future, become educated about the financial world, and learn how to be wise financially – learn how to create wealth by earning interest with your money.

Today's standard of living is higher than ever before.[309] We are living in nicer homes, driving nicer cars, and have more of not only the necessities of life, but more of the luxuries of life than any previous generation. But the sad reality is we are also more in debt, and this debt is financial bondage.[310]

Dr. Clayton is a Professor of History and former Dean of Graduate School. He believes that public and private debt has become the most compelling issue of our day.[311] The second bit of sound financial advice is, *stay out of debt*. Debt is hell; if you want to see what it is like to be in hell, then get into debt. ☺ Financial prison is the best way to describe most debt. Yes, there are things we will likely not be able to pay cash for...our house, our cars, and possibly our education. It is

most often better to buy a house than rent, especially if interest rates are low, so sometimes debt does make financial sense. It might also be better to get through school quickly on loans rather than working our way through school. Sometimes we just have to have reliable transportation and do not have the cash to pay for it...but, if possible, let's not go into debt for a car, and pay cash for school. If you are in debt, pay off your debts that have the highest interest rates first, and those that have the smallest balance first, so you can see the light of *no debt* at the end of the tunnel.

"Interest never sleeps nor sicken or dies; it never goes to the hospital; it works on Sundays and holidays; it never takes a vacation; it never visits nor travels; it takes no pleasure; it is never laid off work nor discharged from employment; it never works on reduced hours...it is as hard and soulless as a granite cliff. Once in debt, interest is your companion every minute of the day and night; you cannot shun it or slip away from it; you cannot dismiss it; it yields neither to entreaties, demands, or orders; and whenever you get in its way or cross its course or fail to meet its demands, it crushes you."

—J. Reuben Clark

Now, after having said all that, let's say a few positive words about debt. Sometimes in business debt is the best thing you can do to secure your financial future and leverage yourself. But be very cautious; evaluate every situation differently, on its own merits. If debt makes the most sense for you and your family, then do it. Protect your family in case something goes wrong. Hope for the best but plan for the worst. Legally separate your family finances from your business finances as much as possible. Set some money aside that cannot be touched no matter what happens. If Donald Trump goes bankrupt on a business deal, do you think he will be living in the streets? Not a chance. Set up a family trust or something where creditors cannot touch at least some of your family assets. It might make sense to set up a corporation or an LLC (Limited Liability Corporation) for every

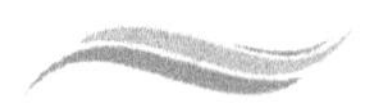

business deal you do, so you have some level of personal protection. You can do this yourself for as little as $50.

Financial stress is proven to cause more divorce than any other single issue in marriage. Close to 80% of all divorces are directly related to financial matters.[312] American's are living off of borrowed money; most live paycheck to paycheck with huge amounts of debt and pay huge amounts of interest on that borrowed money. There is a saying that is a very important principle for each of us to learn, *"Those who understand interest earn it, those who don't pay it!*[313] If you get nothing else from this discussion remember these words. They will bless you throughout your life if you put them to use.

If you have a financial advisor in the family or end up hiring one of our certified financial planners, sit down with them, or online or over the phone, and have them explain more about the Rule of 72. Here's a brief explanation:

The rule says that to find the number of years required to double your money at a given interest rate, you just divide the interest rate into 72.[314] For example, if you want to know how long it will take to double your money at 8% interest, divide 8 into 72 and get 9 years. The rule is remarkably accurate, as long as the interest rate is less than about 20%; at higher rates the error starts to become significant. You can also run it backwards: if you want to double your money in 6 years, just divide 6 into 72 to find that it will require an interest rate of about 12 percent.

Interest Rate	Years to Double
1%	72
2%	36
3%	24
4%	18
5%	14
6%	12

Interest Rate	Years to Double
7%	10.3
8%	9
9%	8
10%	7.2
11%	6.5
12%	6
13%	5.5
14%	5.1
15%	4.8

So why is it important to understand this rule? Because it is really important to understand the principle of compound interest, and that your money will take on geometric growth if you leave it in an interest-bearing account.

"Compound interest is the greatest mathematical discovery of all time."

—Albert Einstein

If you invest a couple hundred dollars a month from the time you are in your 30's into a good interest bearing account, you will have a couple hundred thousand dollars when you retire.[315] This is great, but what's so much better is to invest this same amount in an interest-bearing account from the time you are in your 20's, 10 years longer, and you will end up with over a $million dollars by the time you retire.[316] How could only a few short years of putting a couple hundred dollars a month away make such a big difference? ***Compound interest.*** Taking full advantage of the compound interest growth curve. This is the power of earning interest on your money and growing it over time!

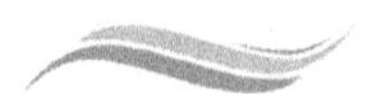

It's like the question of if you would rather have $1,000 a day for 30 days or a penny doubled every day for 30 days...your initial reaction might be to take the $30,000 and run, right? Take a minute to figure it out and you will understand, the penny a day doubled is a *much* better deal. Millions better!

Who understands the principle of compound interest? Most of the wealthy do. This is why they generally do not lose their money. Wealthy people just keep making more. The rich view money as something to earn more money with, not to spend.[317] Poor people generally view money as something to spend, not earn...the exact opposite.[318] Yes, the rich have great lifestyles, but most live well below their means and look at money very differently than the average person. They are always looking for opportunities to invest their money in which are safe, and will yield significant amounts of interest.

If you are earning less than 4% on your money you are going backwards, because this is what inflation has been for the last 30 years. (Source – Bloomberg) We must keep up with inflation or we are going backwards, right? But the sad reality is that most people are paying much more interest on their money than they are making.[319] How smart is this? It's not. Many are so worried about keeping up with the Jones's that they lose sight of what's most important, a secure financial future. The ironic part is we could have so much more than the Jones's if we were a bit wiser with our money. "I want that new car or that nice big expensive house now." That's great, this is the American dream, but what are the costs?

Charles Given's says that two of the biggest wastes of money in our society are:

1. New cars
2. Homes purchased over 30 years[320]

Interest rates on many new cars are really good these days, some even have zero interest, so what's so bad then? The depreciation will

absolutely kill you. What's even worse is spending all that money on a car. New cars are said to lose about half their value the first four years.[321] So if you buy a new car for $20k it is worth $10k after four years. If you buy a car for $50k, it is worth $25k after four years.

Yes, we have to have cars, but what can we do with the money we spend on them? Add interest on to the above total, and include taxes, insurance, gas, and licensing, and we are up around $5-10k per year, or $25k-50k total. How much money would we have today if just 1/4 of that money was put into a good interest-bearing account from the time we bought our first car? You probably don't want to know, and what's a million times worse (literally) is the amount of money we've given up at retirement.

People sell their financial futures for a pot of porridge. It is like people are stuck in high school, and they need to look cool in front of their friends, so they buy a nice new car, so they have bragging rights. Or they just figure they need good reliable transportation and buy into the lie that the only way to get this is to buy new. Maybe you do have money to burn, and a new car is no big deal? It still doesn't make much financial sense. Use that money for something else that will help someone. Buy a car that is at least four years old, so you avoid most of the huge amounts of depreciation. You don't need to skimp on style or features in your car, in fact you can probably buy a lot nicer car, and if you look you can likely find one with hardly any miles on it.

Recently there was a Bentley for sale that sold for about $200,000 new. It only had 12k miles on it, and it was selling for just $29,000. It was 10 years old, but it was in almost perfect condition. Many people that buy these kinds of cars new treat them better than they do their own children. If you like Bentley's, why not buy it? 99% of the people in the world could not tell the difference between this and a brand new one. You can likely drive it for 5-10 years and sell it for about what you paid for it. It you keep the miles low you might even be able

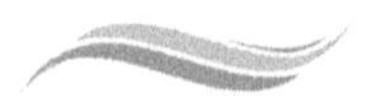

to double your money, and you are driving a Bentley. Someone lost $170,000 on that car, but you can make money on it.

Now, most people do not want to buy a Bentley, mostly because of possible maintenance issues, but listed below are examples of three different types of vehicles, two cars and one truck, that have great reputations and terrific value, if you buy them right: a Land Cruiser, a Corvette, and a Lexus 400 sedan. Obviously, you might not be interested in these, but this discussion will teach general principles that can be applied to all makes and models.

If you have a family; how about 10-year-old Land Cruiser that has only 60k miles on it? The new ones sell for about $100,000. These trucks are built to last; you see them all the time with 200+k miles on them. If you buy a low-mile one for only $10-15k, how badly can you really get hurt financially? You can run up the miles on it and sell it for close to what you paid for it, and you are driving a Land Cruiser.

Or maybe you want a sports car like a Corvette? Why not buy a 10-year-old model, if you look you can find them with low miles (30k or less) and pay in the $10-15k range for them...these are cars that sold for about $50k new. A low mile Corvette might be easier to find than a low mile Land Cruiser because the Corvettes are generally second or third cars, people often sit them in their garages and only drive them occasionally, when the weather is good or for date night. If you buy it for $15k, with only 20k miles on it, you can drive it another 50k miles, then sell it and maybe only lose $2-3k. You can drive a Corvette for 50,000 miles and only spend $3,000! Most Corvette owners lose this much the minute they drive their car off the lot.

How about the Lexus 460 sedan? You can find 10-year-old 460's that have less than 50k miles on them for about $10k. These cars were about $70k new, and the brand-new ones are about $100k. This is one of the best cars ever built. They get 20+ miles to the gallon, are one of the smoothest cars you will ever drive, have V-8's with lots of power, and all the great features like: moon roof, cruise control, Bose

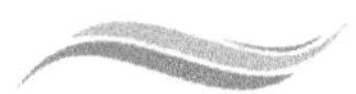

sound system, leather, and heated seats. They are also one of the most dependable cars that have ever been built.

It's just crazy to spend much more than this on cars. Is there much difference in quality, features, or performance between new ones and the 10-year-old models? Not much. Maybe 5%. Does anyone really care that you are driving a 10-year-old Land Cruiser, Corvette or Lexus? Does anyone really know the difference? Most people don't know and don't care. If your family and friends know and are financially educated, they will think you are really smart for buying like you did. If you like the classics, it's hard to lose if you buy them right, because most continually *appreciate*, you are earning money on your car, and you can drive it! If you want attention from your friends, and everyone else, pull up in a 1957 Chevy Bel Air that is lowered, has 18-inch rims, perfect paint and body, and everything is new. If you look you can buy one of these in the mid-$30'-$50's; and make $10,000 - $30,000 on it when you sell it. Or just keep it and enjoy it.

Another great option is to put an electric motor put into a cruiser of your choice, maybe an old T-Bird; with current technology you can get the equivalent of as much as 250 miles to the gallon, if you drive mostly around town.[322] The good life financially doesn't mean boring!

Now, there are lots of problems with acquiring and disposing of electric car batteries, just stay informed and be wise.

Use autotrader.com, cars.com, classiccars.com, or other sites to find the cars/ trucks you want. Just type in whatever kind of car or truck you are looking for and at the click of a button you can search *millions* of listings. You could go down to your local used car dealer and buy an OK car or truck for a certain price, that maybe has 80k miles on it, or you can do a five-minute search on Autotrader.com and find that same car or truck that is in *mint* condition, and only has 40k miles on it; half the mileage, half the wear and tear, for about the same price, sometimes even less. Yes, you might have to take a trip

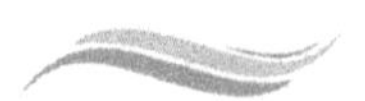

to pick it up or go see it then have it shipped for $1,000, but with the Internet, digital cameras, and Car Fax's (tells the cars history), you can get a really good feel for the car or truck without even seeing it in person. You get the idea. Our computer world is amazing; use it!

Buying homes over 30 years can be a million times worse (literally) than buying new cars. If you take out a 15-year loan on your home you will save tens of thousands, sometimes hundreds of thousands of dollars, and have it paid off in half the time. Yes, your payment will be a little higher, but it will amaze when you find out that it's not that much more, usually only a couple hundred dollars more a month. Often you can make up for the extra couple hundred a month by finding a great deal, building your own home, or buying a fixer-upper, ultimately ending up in a better situation than you could have ever dreamt. It might be better to take out a 30-year loan and just pay ahead on your mortgage or pay ahead on your 10–15-year loan, but *make sure* you tell the mortgage company that you want your extra payment applied to the principle, not the interest. If you don't most often they will just add it like another regular payment where hardly anything goes to the principle. You want to pay off the loan NOT pay interest! By paying ahead you will save thousands every year that can be put into a good interest-bearing account.

After having said all this, there are situations where it is wise to acquire an interest only loan where you pay only on the interest and not on the principle...so, if you kept it for 30 years you would still owe the principal amount borrowed. Why would anyone do this? Maybe you are buying and selling fixer uppers, or taking advantage of what is the best tax break for homeowners out there right now. A couple can make as much as $500,000 every two years on the home they live in when they sell it and pay no taxes.[323] *This is tax-free money!* It's $250,000 if you're single. Many people in the marketplace take advantage of this tax break and build a new home, live in it for two years, and then sell it and do it again. In this situation, where you are

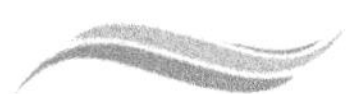

going to sell your home right away, it might make more sense to do an interest only loan, and maybe use the extra money to make the home even more attractive to potential buyers? Sometimes it also makes better sense for tax purposes, or because you can do a better job with your money than whatever interest rate your loan is costing you. But be cautious because it is easy to blow it on useless stuff. The interest only loan is the preferred loan in Europe as it keeps your payments low, so you can live in a nicer home, or just take the extra money each month and invest it in a safe interest-bearing account, or invest it in something really good, so you end up with much more when you retire. Just remember the guiding principle, *earn interest don't pay it.*

This leads us to another important financial discussion. Where do we find a good interest-bearing account? Some would start this discussion talking about mutual funds, and how they have averaged over 12% interest over the last 80 years. But because of our very uncertain economic times, and with wars and rumors of wars ever before our eyes, let's go back and start with the basics or the necessities of life. What are they? Food, clothing, shelter, and transportation. These are the things that make the most sense to have and own, especially in uncertain economic times. People always need a roof over their heads, food to eat, clothing to wear, and a way to get around. Put your money here and it's hard to go too wrong, no matter how bad things get.

Now don't go and sell everything to invest in real estate, or a food company, because you might lose it all if you are hasty and don't know what you're doing. Use your head. Every situation is different and must be evaluated on its own merits.

Unless we have a successful business, real estate might be the best place to put the majority of our money. Real estate across the U. S. typically appreciates about 7% a year, which keeps us above that 4% inflation rate.[324] But if you are smart you will invest in real estate in a great area (location, location, location), and have a killer deal

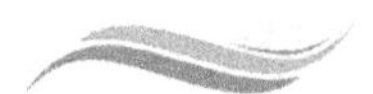

going on, you might earn as much as 20-30% or more on your money a year in real estate. That means if your net worth was $100,000 a year ago, it's $120-130,000 today, or if it was $1 million a year ago, it's $1.2 to $1.3 million today. That's pretty darn good just a year later. Multiply that by a few years and see where you are at! Typically, real estate across the U.S. never goes down in value, even when interest rates have been upwards of 20%. But even when it does go down, like in times of recession or depression, it creates great opportunities for investors. Whatever you do don't get in over your head. Some people borrow up to 100% or more of the value on their homes. Don't live on the edge like this unless you have something else to back it up in case something goes wrong.

In 2009-2020 interest rates were often at a 30-year low. Was this a good time to buy? Yes. Money was cheap. If possible, use times like these to your advantage. Does this mean you go into dreaded debt? Maybe, if you can find a really good deal. Buy low and sell high. During the Great Depression millions of people lost everything, but many also made $millions because they were not living on the edge and had money saved up to invest. So, when things were low, they bought it all up, and then when everything rebounded, they made a fortune. Remember the simple yet profound principle, *buy low and sell high.*

The list can go on and on about what is good and bad to invest in within the food, clothing, shelter, and transportation realm, but just follow the sound principles of investing in things that historically earn huge amounts of interest, and you will not go too wrong, and if you are patient, you will do something really good.

Let's talk now about the importance of having an investment strategy, and an investment portfolio where you spread out your risk; investing in different things so if one thing goes bad, you will still be OK, because you are investing in so many different things.

"If you don't stand for something, you'll fall for anything"

—Alexander Hamilton

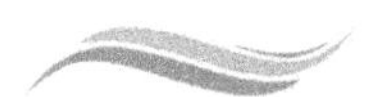

Have a plan that makes sense to you. Don't just live day to day without a plan or nothing you really believe in. Plan your financial future; don't leave it to chance. Here's an example of an investment portfolio strategy:

Personal Investment Strategy

1. Stay out of personal debt as much as possible
2. Earn interest don't pay it.
3. Have an interest-bearing account savings plan (at a good rate of return) and don't touch it until retirement; and set one up for each child too.
4. Set up a college fund for each child.
5. If there's extra money to work with don't put it all in one place, spread out the risk. Like the following:
    a) 5% into food storage (1-year total family supply)
    b) 10% into a bank savings program – Secured by the U.S. Government
    c) 40% into a low-risk investment like: Real Estate
    d) 20% into a medium-risk investment like: Gold or Mutual Funds
    e) 15% into a high-risk investment like: Individual stocks
    f) 10% onto a very-risky investment like: A friend's start-up business

We've talked about debt, interest bearing accounts, and college funds. Let's talk more in depth about what to do with your extra money. Many of you might be saying what, "extra money?" If you don't have any, get some. Follow basic principles of wise money management, and get financially educated, so you know how to make enough interest on your money to have some disposable income. Here's a possible strategy of what to do with your extra money:

a) **Food Storage** – One day food storage for you and your immediate family might be more valuable to you than a two-carat diamond ring on your finger. Not to sound like a radical or pessimist here, but tragedy might strike any of us at any time. If you have food storage on hand you can at least survive until help arrives. A good rule of thumb is to have a year's supply of food on hand for you and your family. You can also save a lot of money on your grocery bill. If you have a place to store your food, like a cold dark cellar or basement, buy things mostly on sale that you can store, say 50%+ off the normal price. Also buy in bulk; you can get things really cheap. Then when you eat rotate your food, eat the food you bought a year ago first, so nothing gets too old. You can cut your grocery bill by 50% by using this simple system. Then put this money into a good interest-bearing account and turn it into millions when you retire or put it into an interest-bearing account for your children, and educate them, so they never have to worry too much about their financial futures.

b) **Bank Savings** - Your interest rate will not be very good, maybe only 1%, but it will be there for you (most likely) in case of an emergency. How often have you needed some extra cash for a really good investment, or a really good deal on something, or just in an emergency, but had none? Be wise. Save 10-20% of your money. The money is secured by the U.S. Government; your money will be as safe as our government. This might scare you deep down inside because our government is tens of $Trillions in debt. So, it's easy to see if everything went really bad, we might not be able to get our money out because there might be a run on the banks... do you remember the movie, It's a Wonderful Life? If this were to happen, we would not be able to get our money out because our money is not in the bank, it is tied up mostly in

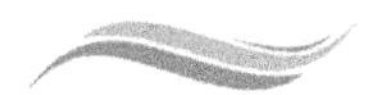

real estate and the stock market, where banks put our money to get a good rate of return, then pay us pennies for using our money. Some think we will never again see days like these where we have a run on our banks but question this logic.

c) **Low Risk** – This is the place it might be wise to put the majority of your extra money, because you likely won't lose it. You will have to be the judge of where a good low risk investment is for you. Some prefer the bank but remember if you're not earning at least 4% on your money, you're going backwards. After 9/11 investors realized the stock market was too risky, so where did many go with their money? Real estate. People across the board recognize that real estate is about as safe as you can get, because, as stated before, people always need a place to live. Real estate has almost always appreciated (time tested), and owning a home is the American dream. But don't get in over your head because your $500,000 home might one day only be worth $100,000-200,000. But if it's paid for, or has a small mortgage, it won't kill you financially. People who live on the edge all around you will be in the panic mode, but you will be fine. This should be the new American dream, owning our own home outright. The other necessities of life are solid too, but likely not as good as real estate. Why? Because they are depreciating assets, and real estate typically appreciates. If you buy and sell cars, you might not be very good at it, but it's really hard to lose too much money because transportation always has value. If you lower the price enough someone somewhere will buy the car. But automobiles are a depreciating asset (unless you have collector cars), so don't hold onto them for long periods of time, and buy the makes and models that will sell, ones that have a good reputation, like Lexus and Toyota. Be careful if you're investing in farming (food) because an unforeseen weather change might wipe out

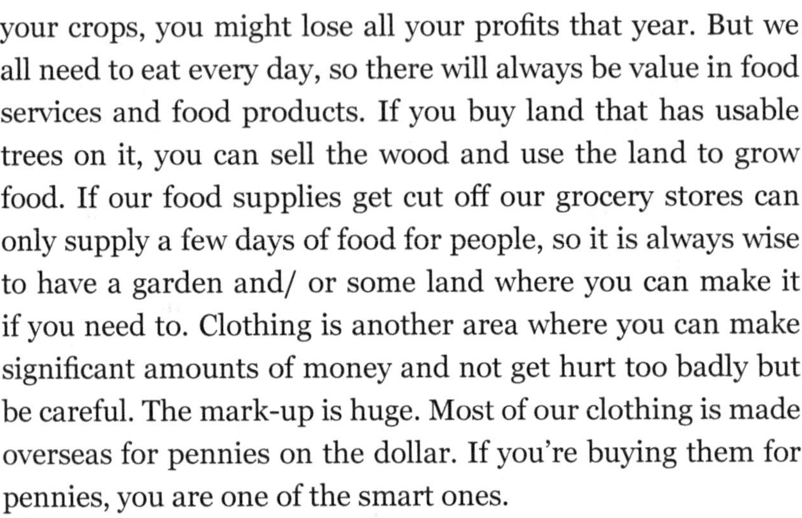

your crops, you might lose all your profits that year. But we all need to eat every day, so there will always be value in food services and food products. If you buy land that has usable trees on it, you can sell the wood and use the land to grow food. If our food supplies get cut off our grocery stores can only supply a few days of food for people, so it is always wise to have a garden and/ or some land where you can make it if you need to. Clothing is another area where you can make significant amounts of money and not get hurt too badly but be careful. The mark-up is huge. Most of our clothing is made overseas for pennies on the dollar. If you're buying them for pennies, you are one of the smart ones.

d) **Medium Risk** – Silver and Gold are great investments; from 2001 to 2009 gold tripled in value.[325] Not too many investments can keep up with this! Too bad we aren't still on the gold standard. Mutual Funds have a good track record. They have earned investors an average of about 12% on their money over the last 80 years.[326] This is remarkable. A good mutual fund manager invests in many different companies and in many different industries...basically the whole stock market would need to fall for you to lose money, which can happen as we've seen. But it will probably rebound and continue to bring investors significant amounts of interest on their money long term. It isn't foolproof. There are risky funds and conservative funds. Like everything else, use caution and be wise. Overall, they do have a good track record, and if you choose a good mutual fund over time, you most likely will stay ahead of inflation and earn a good interest rate on your money.

e) **High Risk** – Buy low, sell high. Why don't people do it? Sometimes people get greedy and think they are about to strike gold, so they throw everything they have at an

individual stock, sometimes buying on margin, and end up losing everything they've worked for their whole lives. They do not follow a wise financial plan that spreads out their risk and makes sense. But most just don't do anything. Individual stocks can be very risky, or they can be more of a medium or low risk investment. Penny Stocks are high risk, but they might have a tremendous return. If you want to invest in individual stocks but want to remain fairly safe, choose stocks that are widely known that will not most likely ever go out of business. Maybe buy them near their 52-week lows and sell them near their 52-week highs. Buy low, sell high... what a concept. Yes, this might take some patience, but it will be hard to lose too much with this agenda, and over time you will likely get a great return on your money. This is what good mutual fund managers do. You can have more fun and not pay their fees by doing it yourself. There are services out there that can help you see the stock's track record and make this process more scientific. Get them and use them. Another good high-risk investment is currency trading. The thing that is cool about it is it is recession proof; you can make money whether the price of the dollar is going up or down. It is good to team up with others that know the industry, have a good record of making money, and will help you...just copy them. Your currency friends might call you in the middle of the night to make a trade, but it is worth it if you're making money!

f) **Very Risky** - Don't put all your money here but do put some. Why? Because financially it might set you up for life. A good example might be a friend that has a great idea for a business but has no money or needs more capital for their start-up business. Help them out for a couple percent of the company. You could be worth $millions from a

two-thousand-dollar investment into a start-up company that makes it long term...yes, most fail, but what if this works? Just one percent ownership could set you up. But be careful, you don't want to throw even a couple $thousand away, because you can use it for something else. Investigate the company, its officers, ideas, etc., thoroughly. Investments that are high risk have the allurement of a craps table, and some throw everything they have at them in the hopes of becoming rich. Don't do it. Your odds might be worse than Vegas. Speaking of Las Vegas, why do people spend so much money there? How do people think they built all those amazing buildings? If you are one of the ones that helped, stop. Eat at their restaurants and enjoy the entertainment, but don't put one penny into gambling. Take advantage of them; don't let them take advantage of you. Be the smart one. It's a black hole and there are so many better uses for your money. People line up in the grocery stores playing the lottery...their optimism is to be admired, but it just isn't very smart. What are the odds of striking it rich? One in a million? If you like the challenge of playing with money, then trade stocks, or buy and sell currency. If you learn some sound investment strategies you can make $millions, and your odds can be really good. Invest in the gambles like a friend's business, that have a much better chance of striking gold, and it is a lot more fun because you can help a friend with a great idea. What goes around comes around. But be wise; don't throw your money away.

"We try to gamble our way into prosperity, and, in the process, we further impoverish ourselves. In 1994 alone, Americans spent 482 billion dollars on gambling – more than they spent that year on movies, sports, music, cruise ships, and theme parks combined."

—Standing For Something

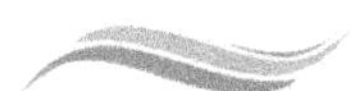

If you have an extra $10,000 this year, don't go blow it on the lottery or on a new car. Maybe take half of that and put it into a solid real estate deal, using it as a down payment on a rental property that has a positive cash flow.[327] Then maybe take $3,000 of that and use it as a down payment on a used car with a really good interest rate, a car that is a little older but is in great shape and has low miles, yet still has a lot of style and the features you are looking for. Then maybe invest another $1,000 in a mutual fund where the only way you will lose is if the bottom falls out of everything. Then with that last $1,000 maybe help your friend who has a great idea but has no money to back it up. Maybe that small investment will turn out to be the thing that allows you to pay off your mortgage and pay cash for everything else? If you lose it, it's OK, you didn't lay that much on the line. This is how WAVE got started. If people just followed some of these basic principles of sound financial planning, they would not be 40 years of age and have a net worth of zero, or be 65 and be dead or dead broke like most Americans.[328]

So many in today's world justify a little sin to get ahead in life, but...

"Dishonesty is like a boomerang. About the time you think all is well, it comes back and hits you in the back of the head."

—H. Jackson Brown

Take these sayings to heart and don't let the temptations of the moment or the dishonest short-term fix overrule your integrity. Nothing is worth that price.

Financial education is the best way to become financially secure and make it possible to have some of the finer things in life. Maybe instead of getting that job that requires the 50+ hour work week, take a job that has a 40-hour work week, if you can find one, and spend some of your spare time learning how to build or repair houses, so you can buy some rental properties, or fixer-uppers and sell them on

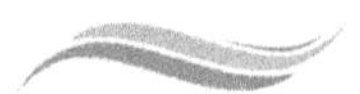

the side. You will be your own boss and it can be really fun. You can get family members involved and make it a family project. You can teach your kids how to work at something productive, skills that will bless them the rest of their lives. Plus, you just might be able to quit working for someone else and do it full-time.

Become a real estate investor or developer. This is where the real money is at. Or, do something else that you enjoy. Maybe start an online business that you can do from your own home, or buy and sell cars on the side. Find a need and fill it. If you can think of something that can be distributed nationally, or internationally, you are likely on a good track. There are a million things you can do, and many of them can be done right out of your own home, so you don't have to be away from your family.

You don't need to cheat, steal, or lie to get ahead. It's amazing how many people are willing to sell their good name, or cheat and steal and lie, for a few more dollars in their pocket. Is their honor really that cheap? Is your soul worth that money you will make off that dishonest deal? Create a legacy for your children and grandchildren to live by.

"No legacy is so rich as honesty."

—William Shakespeare

Make them proud to carry your family name and be your posterity.

If you are interested you can sign up with one of our certified financial planners or personal development coaches, they will help you incorporate these principles of sound financial management into your life. Visit our website at wave4life.com. Take charge of your life, and your financial future, do not leave it to chance. Our coaches can help empower you to develop a solid, realistic plan, one that you feel good about, one that excites you, one that you can and will follow.

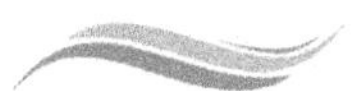

Become financially educated! Don't rely on anyone to tell you what's best. Take advice and counsel, but you become the one that finds the great deals and causes your money to grow. Nobody will ever care as much as you do. So, become educated so you make good decisions. Above all else remember to *earn interest don't pay it.*

DISCLAIMER: Neither tom wright, wave international, nor any of its affiliate companies, divisions, officers, employees, coaches, or independent contractors accept any responsibility, liability, or damages for advice given here. the purpose of this discussion is to teach correct principles of sound financial management so you can personally take responsibility for your financial future and make good choices. these principles are very general and each situation is drastically different. So, it is the sole responsibility of each and every person to determine which advice can and should be applied to their own particular situation, and thus each individual is responsible to make good economic choices and not blame any person or company for money lost. Be very careful with others who profess to know what's best for you in your particular situation. There are many scam artists just waiting to lure unsuspecting prospects in and steal their money, so proceed with caution and *be wise*. Your "financial education" is the key factor for you making good financial decisions. Included is a list of good reading material at the end of this book and would encourage you to make this a lifetime goal, to become financially educated.

QUESTION EVERYTHING?
DAD, HOW LONG COULD WE LIVE ON OUR FOOD STORAGE?
QETommy.com

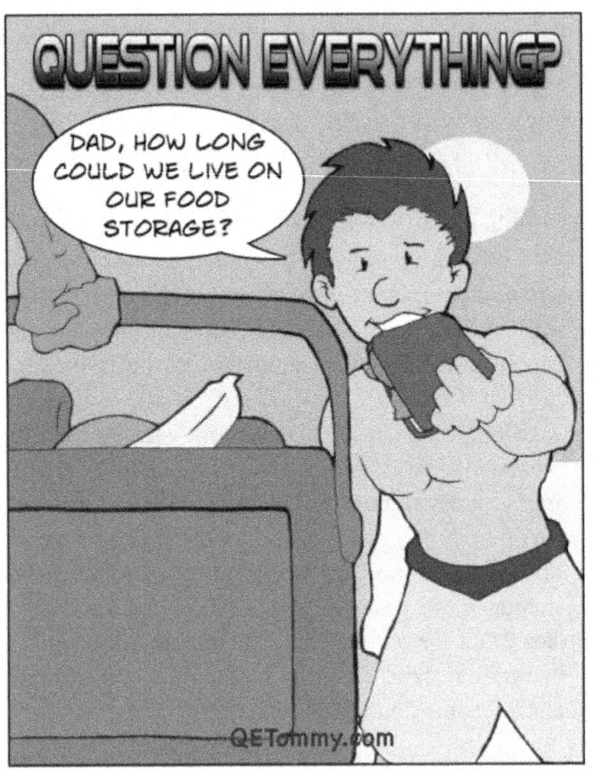

PRINCIPLE #6
Work & Rest & Play!

Find the Balance!

"I know of no more encouraging fact than the unquestionable ability of man to elevate his life by conscious endeavor."

—Henry David Thoreau

There are so many wonderful quotes by so many of the great people in history about the importance of work to achieve our desired results in life. Leonardo DaVinci said, "Oh Lord, Thou givest us everything, at the price of an effort." And Thomas Paine said, *"That*

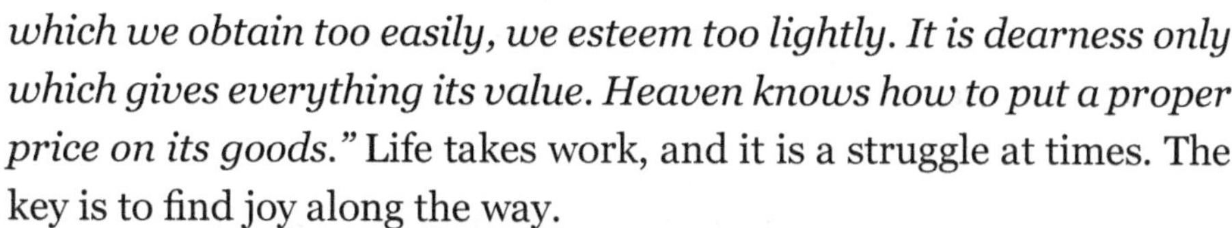

which we obtain too easily, we esteem too lightly. It is dearness only which gives everything its value. Heaven knows how to put a proper price on its goods." Life takes work, and it is a struggle at times. The key is to find joy along the way.

Do not try to do more than you are able, for God does not require that we run faster than we are able.[329] This is where *rest* comes in. If you are tired, rest (The *WAVE*). Cease from being idle, work hard at what you do, be diligent that you might win the prize, and be faithful to the end. "Life by the inch is a cinch, but by the yard it is hard." Work on your goals every day of your life so they are not just dreams. Create your own heaven here on earth.

Be *proactive*. Take charge of your life; don't let it take charge of you. You are the master of your own destiny. Take responsibility. Let God help you be your best self and don't make excuses, rather chose to be valiant.

"Highly proactive people recognize that responsibility. They do not blame circumstances, conditions, or conditioning for their behavior. Their own behavior is a product of their own conscious choice, based on values, rather than a product of their conditions, based on feeling."

—Stephen R. Covey

Commitment is a key factor in our ability to accomplish our desired results. How many people give up right before the blessings flow? How many people give up on their marriage before it gets going? People are swayed by popular opinion and fads of the moment. Many will not work at anything. They move from thing to thing, person to person, looking for happiness, but don't stick with anything or anyone long enough to find success and joy in their accomplishments.

Vision takes the monotony out of life.

"Thought without work is daydreaming;
Work without vision is monotony."

—Thomas Monson

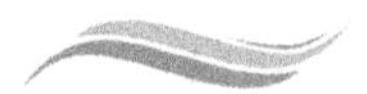

If you know you are in tune with God and His will for your life, you will feel great joy and happiness, and achieve eternal reward in the life to come.

How sad it would be to live a life thinking that when you are dead that is it. No more family, no more spouse or children, no more knowledge or intelligence, no more spirit or body...many people live like this, they really believe this. Can you see how this philosophy would affect their daily decisions? Live for the moment. Do whatever it takes to get ahead. It doesn't matter who they hurt or what they do as long as it benefits them. They might think: why develop relationships? They will end when life is over. Why gain knowledge and intelligence? Just to get ahead in this life. What a sad way to think and live. It takes people away from life's greatest joys. The focus is on this world and the pleasures of the moment, with no thought of God, or an afterlife.

Successful people have vision and keep their dreams alive and well.

"The poor man is not he who is without a cent
but he who is without a dream."

—Harry Kemp

They work through the trials and tribulations of life and keep on keeping on.

When successful people fall, they get back up and back on track. They don't wallow too long in their trials or their lot in life. They move forward and do the best they can do in their present circumstances.

"For the race is not given to the swift or strong,
but those who endure to the end."

—Ecclesiastes 9:11

Success is a journey, not a destination, something very personal. We often judge ourselves, and others, by our material possessions or positions in life, without consideration of progress and personal accomplishment.

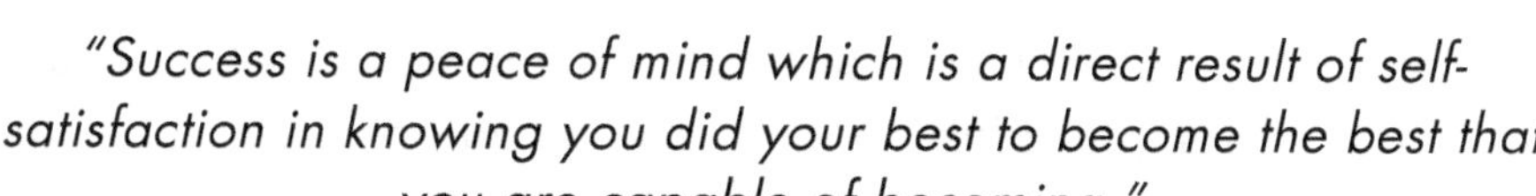

"Success is a peace of mind which is a direct result of self-satisfaction in knowing you did your best to become the best that you are capable of becoming."

—Coach John R. Wooden

Competition can be a good (fun) thing, or it can be destructive. Many people's self-esteem, or what better describes it, feelings of worth, is tied very closely to whether they win or lose on the athletic field, or in whatever circumstance they may be in. This is not good. This is a form of the sin of pride.[330] It comes back to charity (see Principle #3 in Spirit Section). Are we motivated by our love of God and our desire to please Him, and glorify Him, or our desire to have others praise us and glorify ourselves?[331] If you have ever been in the spotlight, it can be very addicting. It feels great to have others tell us how wonderful we are. But we must realize most of this is very superficial and will come and go with the whims of the world.

Our feelings of being on the right track should be based upon our relationship with God, if we are right in His sight. Abraham Lincoln wisely stated, "It is difficult to make a man miserable while he feels he is worthy of himself and claims kindred to the great God who made him." The praises will come and go but we will always feel good about ourselves because we know we are child of a loving Father in Heaven, and we are doing what He wants us to do. Our future is always very bright with God.

Many people achieve their feelings of worth or self-esteem from their appearance.[332] If we do this what happens when we get older and we lose the beauty of youth? Will we not suffer from low self-esteem and think poorly of ourselves? Maybe this is why so many who have been in the spotlight turn to alcohol and drugs when their fame is waning, or when they get older and no longer have the beauty of youth? If we base our value as people on anything other than our relationship with God, we will always be found wanting, and never be

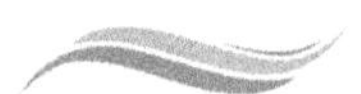

satisfied. How do we ensure that we base our feelings of individual worth on our relationship with God, and not upon other things, like our appearance or the praises of the world? Be a true follower of God and pray for charity with all the energy of heart.[333] Then, and only then, can we have the peace and comfort of knowing we are children of God, we are doing His will, and are motivated by the proper motive (love). There is nothing wrong with looking good, having money, or enjoying life. God wants us to take care of our bodies, and He wants all the best things for us. Let's just make sure we have the proper motivation.

"Our business in life is not to get ahead of other people, but to get ahead of ourselves."

—Maltbie D. Babcock

Competition is fun, if we view it in the proper perspective. **TEAM** - **T**ogether **E**veryone **A**chieves **M**ore. If we work together, we will accomplish more than we could ever do on our own. A great analogy is the study of stresses on 2x4's. If you take one 2x4 and put pressure on it, it will break at about 400 lbs., but if you put (2) 2x4's together you would think it would double to about 800 lbs. before breaking, right? Surprisingly it breaks at about 4x's the pressure, about 1,600 lbs.[334]

This is the way things work if we work together. We can accomplish so much more in life with a good companion by our side. If we have fun with competition, we can inspire one another to accomplish so much more than we could ever do on our own.

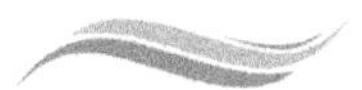

"Teamwork is the ability to work together toward a common vision, the ability to direct individual accomplishment toward organizational objectives. It is the fuel that allows common people to attain uncommon results."

—Andrew Carnegie

Work is the driving force of life. Stay balanced, BodyMindSpirit, and realize there are many forms of work: mental, physical, and spiritual labor. Make work fun and work together with your spouse and family members. This is the way God designed it. Work to make your life great.

In between the work, make sure you're taking time to rest. God himself rested after the 6th day of work...so should we.[335] Rest is an important part of life. Rest at night for the next day, and rest when you get tired. Some say they have no choice--they have to keep going. Who says? Even if we get tired in the middle of a race in the Olympic Games, we can stop and rest if we choose. Now this might not be the best time to do it, but the choice is always ours. There are different ways to be restful. Rest by getting away from your normal day job or activities, whatever that might be. Spend time with your spouse and/or family. Do service activities for others, read a good book, be a true friend...find the balance, BodyMindSpirit.

Many people never really let themselves rest properly or long enough. They are in a constant state of stress and anxiety. Many jobs now-a-days require tremendous amounts of time commitments. The semi-normal 40-hour work week is stretched to 50, 60, and even beyond. Many company heads and managers expect these kinds of hours, or they will find someone else who is willing. This is terrible. It is an attack on the very fiber of our country, our families. Don't do it. Yes, there are circumstances where these kinds of hours are needed. Maybe it's your own business or you have significant amounts of stock in the business, but even then, if these kinds of hours are a constant

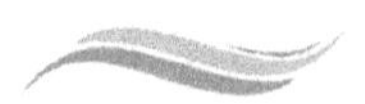

for you find something else to do. Most times these weekly hours are not reflected in compensation.

God expects us to be diligent, but He does not expect us to run faster than we have strength or are able.[336] All things should be done in wisdom, order, and balance. If God himself does not expect this of us, maybe we should not expect this of ourselves, our family members, or other people? Many people do not understand the principle of rest, and others understand it all too well. Balance again is the key. Know when you need to take a break. Know when you are working too hard, too much, or are not balanced...listen, get in tune with God, yourself, and the needs of your family, BodyMindSpirit.

When is the last time you took a vacation? How much sleep did you get last night? Does your spouse always complain you are working too much? When is the last time you went on a date with your spouse? When is the last time you took a child on a date, just you and them? Do you feel tired and run-down? Do you sleep well at night? Do you get headaches often? Is your stomach regularly upset? Do you have health problems related to stress and anxiety? Did you exercise today? Did you eat at least 3-4 healthy meals yesterday? How many hours did you work last week? Did you take time out to meditate, ponder, and/or pray yesterday? Did you take time out to read yesterday? You know when you are out of balance. You know when a change is needed. Listen. Don't ignore the thoughts and feelings.

Some are afraid of change. They have been doing a job for years and are afraid to look for another job where they might have better hours and have more time for themselves and their family. They are afraid to go back to college to get a master's degree so they can get a better job. What if they fail or cannot find another job? Fear is the antithesis of faith!

Others are just in a rut. They have been doing this or that for years and they enjoy it, or they enjoy it enough to not want to make a change, so they just carry on. But deep down they know their life is way out of balance. They know that they suffer and so do their family members because of their choices. But it is not so pressing to force change, just a constant state of stress that they are willing to endure because it is comfortable. Others just figure it is part of life to be stressed out all the time and to not have time with their families and be able to do the things they need to do or would like to do. They figure it's just their lot in life and that there is nothing that can be done. It's just the way it is. *These things are lies!*

Along with God we are the masters of our own souls and destinies. We are responsible for our lives and achieving the balance and proper priorities necessary to be happy and have joy. Take time out of your busy life to rest, relax, pray, meditate, and achieve the balance you desire. So, you can accomplish what you are capable of doing, and have the necessary vitality and strength to carry on in a manner becoming of you, a great son or daughter of God.

One of our important roles here on earth is that of a good friend.

"People who have a close-knit network of intimate personal ties with other people seem to be able to avoid disease, maintain higher levels of health, and in general, deal more successfully with life's difficulties."

— S. Leonard Syme

If you want to learn how to be a better friend to your spouse, your children, and others, read and re-read, the marvelous classic book by Dale Carnegie, *How to Win Friends and Influence People*. It was published in 1936 and has sold millions of copies...and it continues to sell today...this is a classic that has stood the test of time. Books like this will change your life. These are the lessons of history. Dale Carnegie will teach you true principles of healthy living, especially in your relations with your family and other people, which is the most important thing in this life and the life to come. This book has shaped our world.

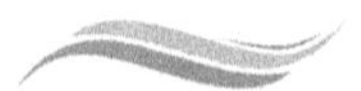

Being a good friend and having good friends is an important part of life. A friend listens, a friend cares, a friend helps...most times with no foreseen reward.

"To have a friend, be a friend."

—Old Saying

A true friend will not encourage you to do anything that is not in your best interest. Of course, all of us are misguided to some degree, but if you truly want to be a friend, you will be a good example to others and yourself.

Example is the best teacher.

A friend does not gossip. Benjamin Franklin's autobiography is one of the most fascinating life stories ever written. In it he explains how hard it was for him to deal with people and all the trouble he got himself into; then he explains how he overcame his problems.

"I will speak ill of no man and speak all the good I know of everybody."

—Benjamin Franklin

This was the key to how he conquered the habit of criticizing others and transformed himself into one of the most able, suave, and diplomatic men in American history.[337]

Of course, if we are parents or are in leadership positions at work we sometimes must explain to our children or employees the consequences of their actions, but we should do it in a loving and kind manner, so they do not look upon us as an enemy or think that we do not love or appreciate them, and try to do it in a way that is requisite for the situation. Usually reproof in private is the best way.

Another important part of a healthy mind is helping others who are less fortunate, being of service to our fellow man. We must impart of our time, talents, and means to helping others if we desire to be

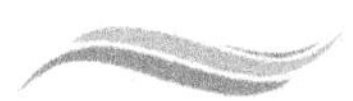

truly happy. Perhaps no other woman in history has done more to relieve human suffering than Florence Nightingale. She was a woman born to wealthy parents but forsook the comforts of wealth to help those in need. She worked with thousands during the Crimean War and spent the remainder of her life (50 years) in both military and civilian hospitals helping those who could not help themselves:[338]

"For those who watched her at work among the sick, moving day and night from bed to bed, with that unflinching courage, with the indefatigable vigilance, it seems as if the concentrated force of an individual and unparalleled devotion could hardly suffice for the first portion of her task alone. Whenever, in those vast wards suffering was at its worst and the need for help was greatest, there, if by magic, was Miss Nightingale."

—Mr. Strachey

Take a break from your work, rest and relax, and look for opportunities to serve those who God has placed around you. Don't wait for them to ask. Discern their needs and reach out with a helping hand. If we are the one that needs the help, we must allow others to help us.

Allowing others to serve us helps lift us up, and it allows the person who gives the opportunity to serve, thus blessing both the giver and receiver.

QUESTION EVERYTHING?
MOM,
HOW COME WE
HAVE TO SLEEP SO
MUCH?
QETommy.com

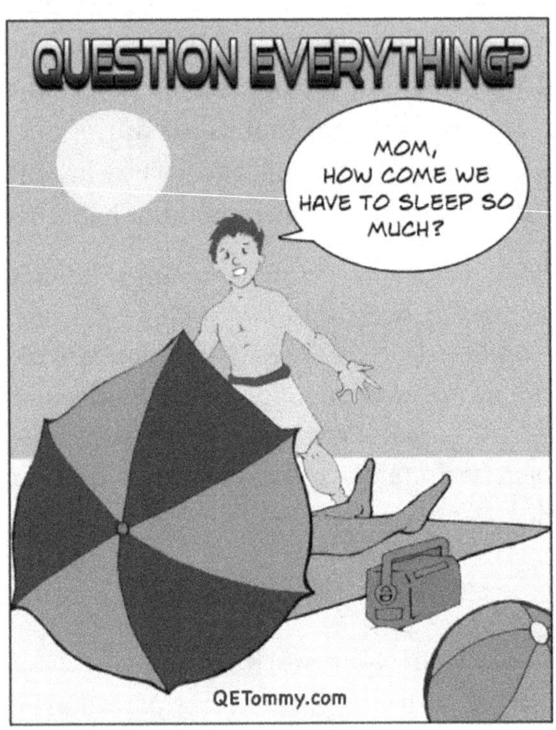

PRINCIPLE # 7
Use a BodyMindSpirit Approach to the Development of Your Mind

Anything less and you go in circles

You are greater than you could ever imagine. We use only 5-10% of our brain power, what are we really capable of? The answer to that simple question is mind boggling, suffice it to say, we can do anything we truly desire in life, if we are right with God.

We must have balance and synergy between all 3 aspects of our nature, BodyMindSpirit, or we will be left to ourselves and achieve much less that we ever could if we have that balance and synergy.

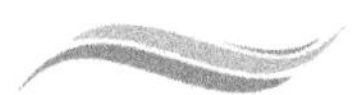

Look to God to find that balance and direction in your life, and He will direct your paths for good.[339] You will never go wrong with Him on your side.

Thank you so much for your time and attention in reading this book! May you use these principles to find more joy and happiness, and achieve more in your life.

We have created many FREE services for you in WAVE because we want to build up a network of good people who are all heading in the right direction. Visit our networking site at, wave4life.com, and take a few minutes to set up your profile. If you are in business, or single, or just looking for some online friends with common interests to have a discussion with, come and visit us.

If you have any great ideas of how to make this book, the TV show, or WAVE better, please write to QETommy@icloud.com with your comments and suggestions. Your comments and suggestions are appreciated.

God bless you in all you do. Now let's move to the most important aspect of our natures, our spirit.

QUESTION EVERYTHING?
MISS KAHAKU,
IF YOU GRADE ON A CURVE
WHAT HAPPENS IF
EVERYONE GETS AN A?
71 + 1107=
QETommy.com

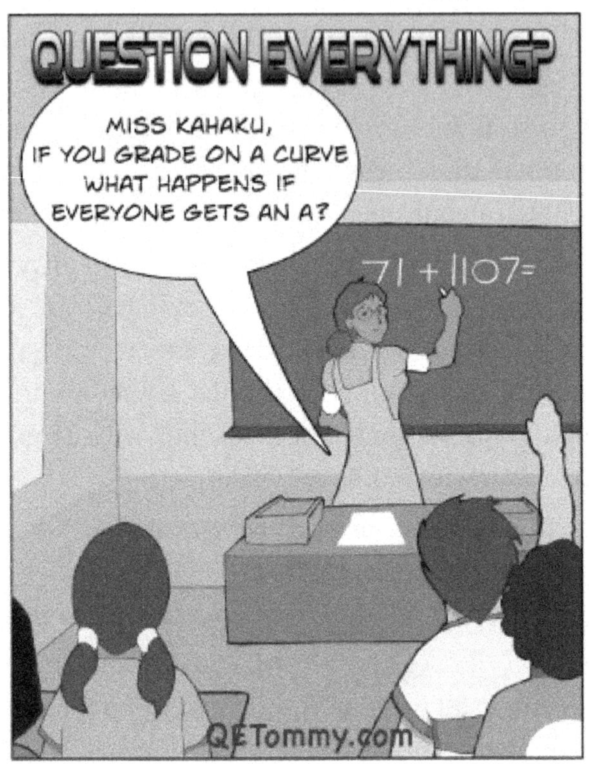

7 Principles of a Healthy Spirit

"If the intrinsic spiritual principles are upheld continually, the physical practices begin to transform one's body and mind. When the training is successfully followed, the metabolic equilibrium developed through the physical practices results in a calmness of mind which, when coupled with the physical power of the body, creates a special condition of vibrant purity."

—Bodhisattva Warriors

INTRODUCTION

The purpose of the 7 Principles of a Healthy Spirit is to help you live a healthy, happy, and productive life. This is the most important section in this book.

We are living in very interesting times. It is a time of great wickedness and corruption, but it is also a time of great righteousness and goodness. There seems to be a greater separation between these two extremes than ever before. Like Charles Dickens said, our days are the best of times and the worst of times.[340] Good people want to see goodness and truth prevail; they want the best for themselves, their families, and the whole human race. This is reflected in our television programs, books, movies, and on the Internet. Oprah Winfrey had a "Remembering Your Spirit" segment on her show, which had a daily viewing audience of about 40 million people.

New York Times' best-selling books like: *The 7 Habits of Highly Effective People*, and *Standing for Something*, talk much about the spiritual side of our nature, the importance of living correct principles of morality, and adhering to spiritual laws of success. Movies such as *Star Wars, Joan of Arc, Tucker, Enchanted*, and *Princess Bride* have a struggle between right and wrong, good and evil, the force and the dark side.

An eternal law that we face as spiritual beings is the law of opposition.[341] We must have opposition in all things to be able to make choices and progress. This might be a simple explanation of why bad things happen to good people.[342] Many do not believe in God

because they see all the bad things happening in our world and say, "if there really was a kind and loving God, He would never let these things happen. There would only be the good and none of the bad. Kind of like the Garden of Eden, a state of peace and paradise."

A good explanation comes in the movie, *Oh God*, where the little boy asks George Burns (God) this very question, "Why do bad things happen to good people?" God pulls out a coin and shows it to the boy and asks, "Have you ever seen a one-sided coin?" Of course not, there is always the other side.[343] This is the law of opposites; in order to have good there must be bad, in order for there to be right there must be wrong, in order for there to be virtue there must be vice. If there were no opposition everything would be a compound in one and vanish away.[344] Remember a kite rises against the wind rather than with it. There must be this opposition in order for us to make choices. Without the ability to choose between good or bad, right or wrong, we would never be able to make choices in life and progress in our journey.[345]

This section, and this whole book, promotes belief in God. The objective is not to offend or alienate anyone, but rather bring to this discussion good and uplifting thoughts and teachings that will help you live a healthier, happier life. No one religion will be promoted, but the Bible and teachings of Jesus Christ will be mentioned. If you are Jewish, Muslim, Buddhist, Hindu or of some other non-Christian religion or belief system, please do not view these words as trying to take away from your faith, rather see if they might be able to add something to it.[346] In a provocative Wall Street Journal article the author shared this insight:

"As we gather...to celebrate the most famous holiday of our long-dominant religious faith, the very idea of religion finds itself under siege. The word of God...dare[s] not be heard in the nation's schools. The crèche cannot be erected on public property; for the first time since the conversion of Constantine, the state has outlawed the

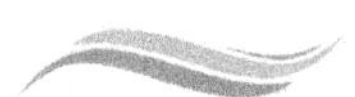

display of Christian symbols. Meanwhile schools distribute condoms, even over the objections of parents...Christianity has instructed us on moral issues for two millennia, and Judaism longer still. With or without personal faith, we have been living off this capital... Rather than denigrating Christianity and religion in general, socially conscious elites ought to be asking what the religious impulse can teach us, and how amid the winds of modernity we might start to replenish the stock of moral guidance it bequeathed us."[347]

In the *New York Times* best-selling book entitled, *Standing for Something*, the author writes: "There is something reassuring about standing for something, and knowing what we stand for. For men or women who are true to themselves, and to the virtues and standards they have personally adopted, it is not difficult to be true to others. Those who are committed to, and have patterned their lives after, a Higher Power need not rely on public opinion, which is often blatantly skewed.

Here is the answer to the conflicts that beset us. Here is the answer to the evils of pornography, abortion, drugs, and the squandering of our resources on evil pursuits. Here is the answer to the great epidemic of litigation that consumes time, saps our financial strength, and shackles our entrepreneurial spirit. Here is the answer to tawdry politics that place selfish interests and pursuits above the common good.

Let all houses of worship ring with righteousness. Let people everywhere bow in reverence before the Almighty who is our one source of true strength. Let us look inward and adjust our priorities and standards, recommitting ourselves to time-honored virtues that embrace right and shun wrong. Let us look outward in the spirit of the Golden Rule. Let us work tirelessly to defend and strengthen the family, which is the fundamental unit of society."[348]

This approach will scare off a few, but most (92%) here in America

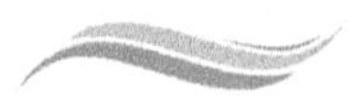

do believe in God;[349] and most also recognize the value of Christ's teachings, even if they don't accept Him as the Savior of the world.[350]

So, our Heavenly Father and Jesus Christ are left in the equation, rather than leaving them out. It's very difficult to talk about a healthy spirit, with honesty and truth, and not mention God. Many beat around the bush and disguise what they are saying, but God is the source of the knowledge and strength of these words, and this fact is freely acknowledged. However, as this book enters other countries around the world these principles will be modified, so as to not offend the people or the countries this book enters. You are getting the "uncut" version here.

If you remember nothing else from this book; remember our UNLIMITED POTENTIAL as spiritual beings.

"We are not human beings on a spiritual journey; we are spiritual beings on a human journey."

—Stephen Covey

The Holy Scriptures repeatedly tell us that we all have unlimited potential as sons and daughters of God.

"I have said, ye are gods; and all of you are children of the most high."

—Psalms 82:6

Do we believe it? Have we received a sure witness or conviction that this is true?

Some might think that if we really do have unlimited potential, and only use a small part (5-10%) of our brain[351], why is it so hard to overcome bad habits, or for a person to take themselves out of the slums, or overcome a negative way of life that we have grown up with? If we really are sons and daughters of God, and we can do anything in this life and in the eternal worlds to come, why is life so hard?

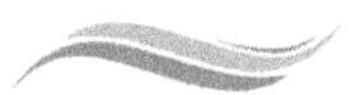

A simple answer might be life is supposed to be this way.

But as we will discuss, we are often the ones that make it this way. We are what we think about. You are the sum total of all your thoughts. Hopefully this isn't a scary thought. The law of attraction is true[352]; we attract to our lives what we send out. If you think life is hard, it is. If you think life is beautiful, it is.

"If you think you can or can't, you're right."

—Henry Ford

Let's also consider that each of us has a specific mission or purpose in life. Not everyone can become President of the United States, even if we all firmly believe we can, and work hard to achieve it, but that doesn't mean we cannot overcome a bad habit or do what we really want to do in life. Deep down inside of you there are thoughts, feelings, and desires that are specific only to you. You have a special purpose in life, and more than one. Ultimately you can do anything you want to do, for the power is within you.

Some important things are left out of this discussion that are not appropriate for a book about healthy living, either because of limited space, or just because of the focus. Please don't judge these words too harshly. There is no apology for this book, God has been very supportive of the effort, but know it isn't perfect, and that it will get better over time. Write to; qetommy@icloud.com with your comments and suggestions. Your comments and suggestions will be taken very seriously. Fair enough? Then let's get started.

QUESTION EVERYTHING?
LANI,
HAVE YOU NOTICED A
KITE RISES AGAINST
THE WIND?
QETommy.com

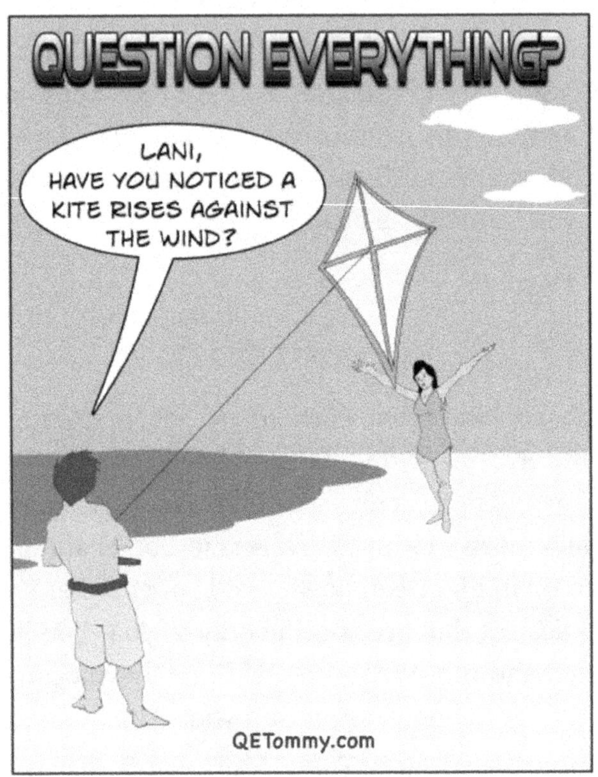

PRINCIPLE # 1
Look To God

He can make a whole lot more of your life than you can

If we look to God, He will bless our life and do a much better job of directing our path than we can.

"The Lord works from the inside out. The world works from the outside in. The world would take people out of the slums. Christ takes the slums out of people, and then they take themselves out of the slums.

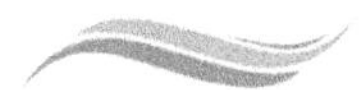

The world would mold men by changing their environment. Christ changes men, who then change their environment. The world would shape human behavior, but Christ can change human nature."

—Ezra Taft Benson

God loves you perfectly.[353] He is aware of your *every* thought.[354] He knows the deepest desires of your heart and sees all your actions. If He notes the fall of the sparrow (Matthew 10:29, 30), would He not be aware of you? Matthew records the fact that He even knows the numbers of hairs on our heads.[355] Why do we not believe this at times? Maybe it's because we lack faith? What exactly is faith? Faith is belief in things that are not seen but are true (Heb. 11:1). When we lack faith, we may feel like we are not loved, like nothing we do matters. We might reason that God has too many others to worry about, why would He be concerned about little old me? As the writer of Proverbs said, "What is man that thou art mindful of him?" (Psalms 8:4) Paul the Apostle responds by saying "we are the offspring of God." (Acts 17:29) We are His children, and He loves each and every one of us perfectly. God will do anything He can, respecting our free agency, to help us progress and be like Him.[356] Just like our earthy parents love and care for us, our Heavenly Father loves and cares for us, but all the more because He is perfect, so he can love and care for us perfectly.

Without this ability to make choices (freedom of the will), we would not be able to progress.[357] If we were forced to do the right things, we would never grow, because we would never have the ability to fail or succeed. War, murder, abuse, starvation, etc. are terrible, terrible things. We should do everything in our power to stop the bad by promoting all the good that we can in our society. God desires all the best things for each and every one of us. He wants us to be happy, have joy in this life, and eternal life (with Him) in the world to come.

Life isn't fair. It is not meant to be that way. Why do so many of the best people this world has ever known suffer so much? Sometimes even death because of others? One of the great movies of the 25 years

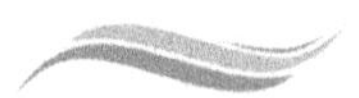

is *Joan of Arc* (the PG one). What an amazing story of a glorious young woman. Good and righteous people are often misunderstood, especially if they do not have the powers to be behind them.

"Blessed are they which are persecuted for righteousness' sake: for theirs is the kingdom of heaven. Blessed are ye, when men shall revile you, and persecute you, and shall say all manner of evil against you falsely, for my sake. Rejoice, and be exceedingly glad: for great is your reward in heaven: for so persecuted they the prophets who were before you"

—Matt.5: 10-12

Life is not easy but with God's help our burdens can be made light.[358] God is perfectly just, merciful and kind, if we have been unfairly dealt with in this life eventually all things will be made right. If we have suffered unjustly, it will be made right either in this world or in the world to come.[359] They can hurt our bodies, call us names, and mock us, but they cannot take away our self-respect and our belief in God.

Some people despise this philosophy. Many think it requires too much faith. But what are the alternatives? Curse God and wish to die? Live without God in the world? Take vengeance into our own hands and suffer the rest of our lives for that vengeance?

"Vengeance in mine, I will repay, saith the Lord."

—Romans 12:19

Our calling is to forgive all people.[360]

We are to follow the Master and live as He lived, so that we can have peace in this world and eternal life in the world to come. Does this mean we should let offenders go free? No, because they might harm someone else. It just means that we should not hate anyone. Hate their evil actions yes but love all people.

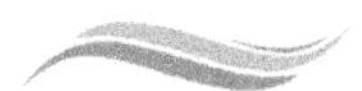

"Love your enemies, bless them that curse you, do good to them that hate you, and pray for them which despitefully use you and persecute you."

—Matt. 5:44

If you carry hate inside you, it will destroy you. Let us follow the higher road, let God fight our battles, let Him be our strength and our song.

Life is hard if we fight it alone. The Savior said,

"Come unto me, all ye that labor and are heavy laden, and I will give you rest. Take my yoke upon you and learn of me; for I am meek and lowly of heart: and ye shall find rest unto your souls. For my yoke is easy and my burden is light."

—Matt.11: 28-30

You can see God's light in people's faces. (Matt 28:3) Some people have tried to do it alone, and it shows. Some people have lost their light. The light they were born with is almost non-existent; they are barely living. Others shine like the noon-day sun. (Rev. 1:16) You can tell just by looking at them that they are good people; they are happy, bright, and alive. They have a sparkle in their eyes and a bounce in their step that only comes from righteous living and casting their burdens upon the Lord. Which side will you be on? Why make life any harder than it has to be?

Look to God. He can do so much more with your life than you can. Pray, seek His guidance, read the scriptures, hear His word, and seek His face.

"Blessed are the pure in heart for they shall see God."

—Matt. 5:8

This scripture means exactly what it says; we can literally see God, and converse with Him, as one-man converses with another. Yes,

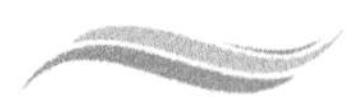

here in this world, before we die. Was this not what the prophets of old did? Why not us? God is no respecter of persons, and He is the same yesterday, today, and forever.[361] We just need to live in accordance with the principles that govern this greatest of all blessings.

Whatever your position or lot in life God will be there for you. Maybe not in the way we always plan, but He has promised us that He will answer our prayers.

"Ask, and it shall be given you; seek and ye shall find; knock, and it shall be opened to you: for everyone that asketh receiveth; and he that seeketh findeth; and to him that knocketh it shall be opened. Or what man is there of you, whom if his son ask bread, will he give him a stone? Or if he ask a fish, will he give him a serpent? If ye then, being evil, know how to give good gifts unto your children, how much more shall your Father which is in heaven give good things to them that ask him?"

—Matt. 7:7-11

So, if righteous living is an easier way to live, if we will be happier in this life and receive eternal reward in the life to come, why do we ever make bad choices, choices that take us away from God and move us toward the Adversary? Temporary insanity.

There is often much pleasure and immediate gratification in sin, but there is no lasting happiness.[362] Sexual immorality is so prevalent in our society. It is hard sometimes to see why is so wrong with sexual relations before marriage and lack of fidelity after marriage. It destroys the very fiber of our being.

People nowadays many times live with a partner, or several, before marriage. Or sometimes choose to never marry. Many times, mocking those who don't, and say something like, "How can you really know what a person is like, or if you are really compatible, unless you live with them first?" The reality is if we keep God's commandments, we will have a much greater chance of a successful relationship than if we don't.

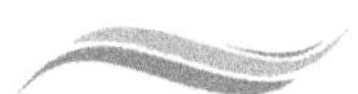

"According to a 1997 nationwide survey, divorce is 32 percent more likely among those who engaged in premarital sex than it is among the general population. And almost three times as many separated or divorced Americans have committed adultery, compared to the general population. Further, 82 percent of adults who rate their marriage as "very strong" (9 or 10 on a 10-point scale) did not engage in premarital sex. This should not surprise us. Immorality is a breach of integrity of the highest order. On the other hand, those who have demonstrated sexual purity are also likely to have cultivated other moral virtues that contribute to the success of any relationship, particularly marriage. Each of us has the capacity to control his or her own thoughts and actions. This is part of the process of developing spiritual, physical, and emotional maturity."

—Standing for Something

No marriage will stand the test of time and bring true joy and happiness to any individual who is cheating on their partner. Just think about it logically, would anyone argue that your relationship with your partner is going to be best if you think only about them? If you are constantly thinking about past relationships, people of the opposite sex at work, etc., you will never be the kind of spouse you could be if you were faithful in thought and deed.

Marriage is a sacred covenant before God and was instituted in the beginning of time in the Garden of Eden.

"Therefore, shall a man leave his father and his mother, and shall cleave unto his wife: and they shall be one flesh."

Gen. 2:24

Feel sorry for individuals who really believe they will be happier by cheating on their spouse and be thankful that you do not. Yes, it might be pleasurable for a moment, but if you give in to those desires it will destroy the trust between you and your spouse, and you will never satisfy those desires you have if you try to do things your way. If the desires God has placed in you are misused, they become insatiable, meaning you will never be satisfied if you do not use them the way God intended.[363] You will always be looking for the bigger and better thrill. After many years you will look back at your life and wonder how you ended up where you are, alone and miserable. God's commandments are there to bless our lives, not hold us back from a fullness of joy. There is a great illustration that helps put this principle in better clarity. Here it is:

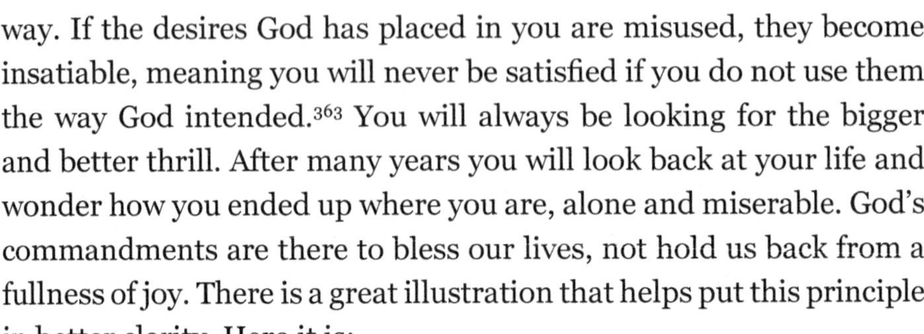

Wickedness never was happiness.[364] This seems to be a hard lesson for most of us to learn, but the evidence is overwhelming. Satan's Plan may seem like total freedom; do whatever it takes to get ahead, lie, cheat, steal, commit adultery, etc. But the end result is total bondage, to our appetites and passions, and the sorrowful results of our choices, and eternal damnation, meaning we cannot continue to progress. Gods Plan, in comparison, might seem restricting; keep the 10 Commandments, no sex outside of marriage, don't lie, cheat, steal,

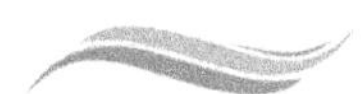

or smoke, but the glorious result is perfect freedom. Freedom from disease and the effects of bad choices, long and lasting relationships, and God's blessings to develop our talents, bless other's lives through honoring Him, and eventually eternal life with God. Even if we don't believe in God and the afterlife, we should be able to see the logic and blessings of keeping God's commandments.

Where there have been problems, there is forgiveness. We have all made many mistakes.

"There is no man that sinneth not."

—1 Kings 8:46

Not one of us has ever lived a perfect life. There is only ONE who has ever done that, He who was slain for the sins of the world.[365] Come to God and you will be forgiven.

Saith the Lord: "Though your sins be as scarlet, they shall be white as snow; though they be red like crimson, they shall be as wool."

—Isaiah 1:18

Often it is assumed that physical or body appetites and passions make us behave a certain way.[366] We might hear the comment, "My body made me do it." The body is element and element by nature is obedient.[367] When God commands the elements, they obey. The same holds true for us. The body obeys the spirit, not the other way around.[368] A logical way to understand this is to realize that the power to choose resides in the spirit. Element is acted upon whereas spirit acts. Element has no power, no capacity to choose, no agency. Agency resides with the spirit.[369]

Of course, we have physical appetites, but that doesn't mean the body acts independently of the spirit. When the spirit joins with the body, this added element gives the spirit a wider range of choices. One of those "new" choices is in the realm of physical appetites. What is occurring is not a battle between choices by the body and choices

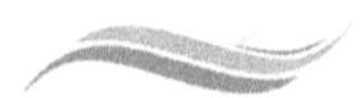

by the spirit. What is occurring is a refinement of the spirit as it learns to deal with the added physical element. If the spirit does not elevate the body beyond base desires, or in other words, gives in to worldly temptations, it may seem that the body is actually in control. All it really means is that the spirit is operating at the basest level; it is not living up to its potential.[370]

If one reads through the creation of the world as recorded in Genesis, the first book of the Bible, it is very apparent that our bodies were created from the dust of the earth and when God commands the elements obey. Our bodies were given to us as a great blessing, a way for us to progress and reach our eternal destiny, and thus should be taken care of in the best possible way.[371]

Some view us on the same plane as the animals. Although some humans do act like animals, animals cannot reason. Their brain waves and mental capacities are far below even the simplest human.[372] We are clearly above any animal, no matter how well trained or advanced they may be. We use only a small percent of our mental capacities, about 5-10%.[373] Those who use only slightly more than the norm accomplish amazing things in life. If Albert Einstein only used 15% of his mental capacities, what could we do if we used 30% or 50%?

We idolize men like Albert for how smart they are, but do we consider that we have the capacity to outdo them by many-fold? Do you believe God would bless us with these great capacities and not let us fully develop them? Is God just playing with us? This doesn't make any logical sense. Christ said if we had faith as the grain of mustard seed, we could move mountains.[374] He also said nothing is impossible to him that believeth.[375]

Reason would teach us that one day it is possible to have full use of all our mental, physical, and spiritual abilities. Ours is a time for testing, and learning – discovering how to grow into our marvelous capacities. We are greater than we could ever imagine. Let us think more on these things instead of putting limits on ourselves and our

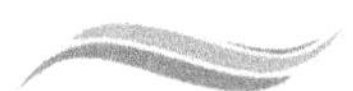

abilities; thinking of ourselves and others to be less than we really are, sons and daughters of God with unlimited abilities.

"The Spirit itself beareth witness with our spirit, that we are the children of God: And if children, then heirs, heirs of God, and joint-heirs with Christ; if so be that we suffer with him, that we may be also glorified together."

—Romans 8:16, 17

God has a special plan for each and every one of us. The movie *Simon Birch* really drives home the point that, "we all have a special purpose here on earth," we all have a reason we were born, certain talents we need to develop, specific things we need to do.

How do we discover or know what we were born to do and capable of doing here on this earth? Or know when we are off track, or maybe just going through tough times where we need to grin and bare it, and continue our course? Here's a list of 3 basic ways:

1. **In Tune with God** - We must be in tune with our Heavenly Father and His will for our lives. We must not be swayed by popular opinion or the cares of the world; His Spirit must guide us. We can know where we stand in His sight. Yes, it might not be easy, and it takes effort, but the price is worth the comfort and peace which will come into our lives as we live in accordance with His will, and are consistent with the Lord.

One way to see if we are living in accordance with God's will for our lives is to...

"...be such a man and live such a life, that if every man were such as you, and every life like yours, this would be God's paradise."

—Phillip Brooks

We have been given our conscience, so we know if what we are doing is right or wrong.[376] But remember, this marvelous

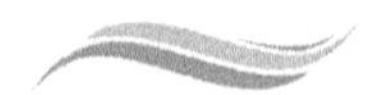

instrument can become dull and will not work properly if we continue in our wayward acts. We must come unto God if we hope to be in tune with Him. We cannot be out of line with God and in line with anything else that is good. We either love God or we love Satan. Will we be as Cain who loved Satan more than God?[377] Or be as all the righteous people who love God more than Satan? The choice is ours. May we be on the Lord's side.

2. **Keep the Commandments** - God has given us the 10 Commandments to guide us in the ways of happiness and peace.[378] Read through the 10 Commandments, become familiar with them, hang them up in your room, memorize them, and keep them. Remember, these are given to us to bless our lives and set us free. When we live in accordance with God's laws our lives will have more freedom, not less. We will be free from guilt, the sorrow of sin, the punishment of the sinner, hopelessness, and a life of mediocrity. We will grow from grace to grace, be happy, have joy, be all that we can be, and eventually be blessed with perfect freedom and eternal life.
3. **Seek Revelation** - Another way to determine if we are living in accordance with God's will for our lives is to seek inspiration and revelation through prayer and scripture study. Heavenly Father will speak to you personally through His Spirit.[379] These personal revelations will be in accordance with the words of the prophets but will be spoken to you personally. God has a special plan for each and every one of us. We all have a special purpose here on earth, a reason we were born, certain talents we need to develop, specific things we need to do. God will communicate to each and every one of us through prayer and inspiration, if we come unto Him. This revelation might not always be in accordance

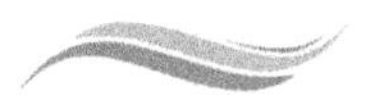

with popular opinion or even reason, for God works by faith, and faith can move mountains. So, don't fear the criticism of others, fear God, for...

"He who fears criticism is hopeless. Only those who do things are criticized. To hesitate for fear of criticism is cowardly."

—Thomas Jefferson

If God has spoken to you personally and you know what you are doing is in accordance with His will, by all means keep the faith. Keep moving forward and you will receive the reward. It may not come in the way you plan or desire, but the blessings will flow.

QUESTION EVERYTHING?
DAD, HOW COME WE USE ONLY 5% OF OUR BRAINS?
QETommy.com

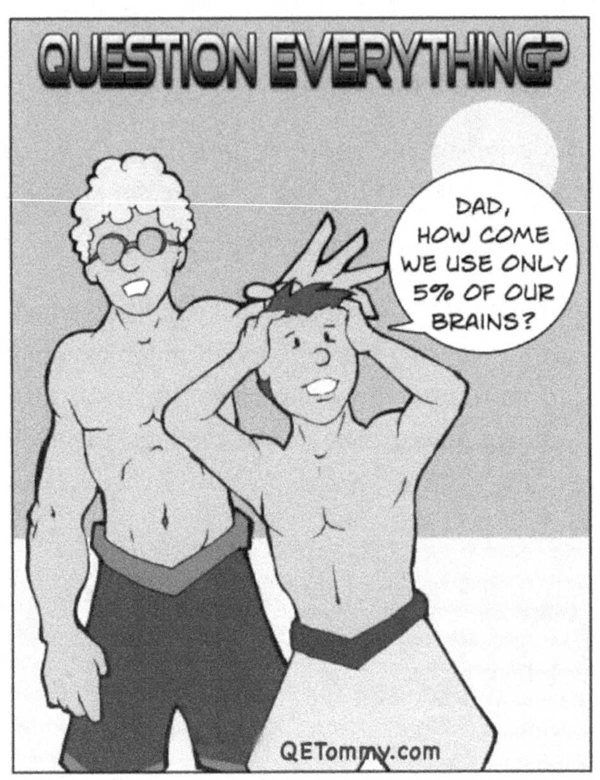

PRINCIPLE #2
Realize Your Potential As A Human Being
The worth of souls is great!

You have unlimited potential, no matter who you are or what you do.[380] If you are a bum on the streets, or the wealthiest man in the world, your potential is the same, limitless. Why? Because you are a begotten son or daughter of God, "if a son [or daughter], then an heir of God through Christ (Gal 4:7). God is your Father. You were created in His likeness and image. The earth you stand on was created for YOU; the beasts of the field, the fowls of the air, every herb in the

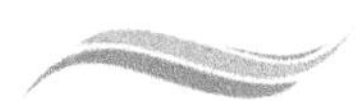

season thereof, and every fruit in the season thereof, it was all created for you and your eternal progress.[381] God's work and glory is to bring about our eternal life.[382] Eternal life means eternal progression and life forever with God.[383] This is our destiny, the purpose of our existence.

Why do we talk about all this in a "healthy living" book? Because if we do not understand our potential as spiritual beings, it is very hard for us to overcome the stumbling blocks that are put in our paths. If you really understand your unlimited potential, the stumbling blocks will become stepping-stones. It will be so much easier for you to unleash your unlimited potential because you will come to know and understand that deep down you are greater than you could ever imagine. Those things that hold you back will begin to seem insignificant, and you will be able to push through those obstacles and do amazing things with your life.

Our bodies are sacred, glorious, and beautiful. We came here to earth to make choices and receive this mortal tabernacle called our body; and then to present our bodies as a living sacrifice, holy, to God.[384]

Some people view the body as evil, something that will be discarded after this life.[385] Yes, we will be separated from our bodies for a time after we die, but then we will receive the glorious resurrection the Savior made possible through His atonement and the power He had over death. All of us will receive a glorified resurrected body and be able to continue to perfect ourselves through time and eternity, along with our spouses and children.[386] Christ broke the bands of death so that we might live.[387] He did not discard His body after death. He was resurrected and showed His body to His apostles and others. If we are, "heirs of God, and joint heirs with Christ" (Rom 8:17), then why would we be any different than what Christ was like after his resurrection? We will all receive a glorified resurrected body just like Christ and live forever with our body just like God and Christ do.

We will live as they live and do as they do; we will have full use

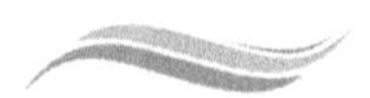

of all our God-given powers, if we are true and faithful to Christ and His teachings.[388]

This is our *mission*, if we choose to accept it, and it isn't impossible. It is within the grasp of every individual who has ever lived upon the earth, or who will yet live. You may ask, but if everything is predicated upon our faith in Christ and His teachings, what about all those billions of people who do not believe in Christ, or haven't even heard of Christ, or who have died not knowing anything about him? There will be a time in the next life, before the final judgment, for everyone to hear the truth and either accept it or reject it.[389] Then the playing ground will be made level, everything that was not fair or right in this life will be made right. But that is no excuse for us who have been taught the truth of these things now, for where much is given, much is expected. (Luke 12:48)

The Lord has promised He will not allow us to be tempted beyond our ability to endure if we are watchful and prayerful. (Matt.26: 41) God's plan is not a plan of failure; it is a plan of success. Satan will try to discourage you and make you think all is lost if you have done this or that wrong, or make his way appear much more fun and exciting. Don't listen to him. He is telling you lies. He is the father of lies and he will carefully drag you down to hell. Will you let him? You are in control. Lean on the Lord; love the Lord with all your heart, might, mind and strength, and He will fight your battles.

Let's talk a bit more about our glorified resurrected bodies. It is really important to understand this point, because each of us needs to understand our marvelous potential. Once created as a spirit, you became a unique individual.[390] Your body looks the same as your spirit.[391] There is no way to lose your individuality, to lose the self that you are. You never become someone else. We will not be reincarnated, but when we die our spirits and our bodies will be separated for a time, then eventually be reunited again (resurrection), and in that state we

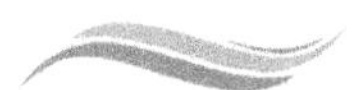

will live forever, with our bodies and our spirits once again together as one. This is what happened to Christ. He died, and His body was placed in the sepulcher, and after three days His spirit once again joined His body and He appeared to many. To some who thought He was only a spirit, Christ said the following:

"Behold my hands and my feet, that it is I myself: handle me, and see; for a spirit hath not flesh and bones, as ye see me have. And when he had thus spoken, he shewed them his hands and his feet. And while they yet believed not for joy, and wondered, he said unto them, Have ye here any meat? And they gave him a piece of a broiled fish, and of a honeycomb. And he took it and did eat."

—Luke 24:39-43

Clearly Christ has a body of flesh and bones as tangible as man's, and now He is a glorified resurrected being, and we will also be resurrected because of Christ.[392] Resurrection means the joining of our spirits and our bodies in a glorified state, never again to be separated.[393] Christ was the first person to ever live who was resurrected, and He made this great blessing possible for all of us.[394]

So, our bodies are not evil, something to be discarded after this life, they are as eternal as our spirits, and are therefore a great blessing to our lives.

Some might think, well, if we are going to receive a glorified resurrected body in the next life, what does it matter how I take care of my body in this life? To which the best response might be; does anything else in life work this way? Do we ever get something for nothing? It makes sense that at some point we must figure out how to take good care of our physical bodies, whether in this life or the next, if we want to reach our full potential. Plus, we must take good care of our bodies to have a good quality of life here and now.

If we really understand this and have proper gratitude, we should be *internally* motivated to take the best possible care of our bodies,

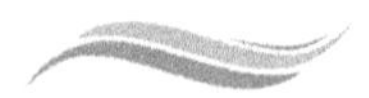

minds, and spirits. We won't need to put a picture of Angelina Jolie or Brad Pitt on our mirrors for motivation. As we come to know and appreciate the fact that we are a child of God, that we have unlimited potential, and that our bodies and spirits will live forever, and are the key to our eternal progress, we will be highly motivated to take the best possible care of our whole selves, BodyMindSpirit.

Even today with organ donations and transplants, these do not alter our eternal selves. When we are resurrected not so much as a hair of our heads will be lost...this is a comforting thought for some.[395] If there are physical impairments, they will be made whole.[396] Because of the glory that will attend us in this resurrected state, the most plain looking people will be more attractive than the most beautiful people here in this life.[397] If God is perfect, how could it be any other way? Christ was not a comely man, people did not desire Him because of His appearance, but now in His glory He is more desired than they all.[398]

Our present view of life is so limited, but one day we will see all things. But until then we must all live by faith. Faith is belief in things that are not seen which are true. (Heb 11:1) We must search out truth; pray about it to make sure it is true, then live by it so we can be made free. (John 8:32)

The more we live according to true principles, the more we are able to express the person we really are.

This might not seem true, but it is. The more we live according to true principles, the more power, individuality, righteousness, and oneness with God we will have in our lives. Often, we do not hear about the lives of the obedient and faithful, because they do not boast or cause undue attention to come their way. If they do seek the limelight, it is to build God's kingdom here on earth, and to glorify Him, not themselves. They do quiet acts of kindness and love that are often only known by those they serve. They follow the life of Christ and do what He would do if He were there in their place. Is Christ one

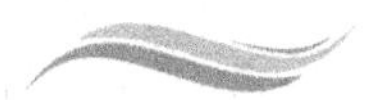

of a kind? Of course, He is. Is He different than all the rest? Yes. If we desire to be different, we will follow Christ and do the things that He did. Then, and only then, will we truly be our own individual selves.

According to the stirring document entitled, Family: A Proclamation to the World, gender is eternal.[399] Many try to confuse this truth by teaching that gender is socially constructed. But if we really take a look at the human race, we can plainly discern that there is a difference between males and females. In the book, *Men are from Mars and Women are from Venus*, many truths are set forth that help us to understand the differences between the genders.

Some people are born in-between the sexes, their X and Y chromosomes are out of balance for either male or female, and as a result they manifest both genders in their reproductive organs. So, some might say, if gender is eternal, how do you explain these people, or those who feel like they were born the wrong sex? This is in God's hands, but they will be either male or female throughout eternity.

Nobody is perfect physically. We all have things about us that will be made right in the next life. We might have scoliosis (curvature of the spine), or unsightly birthmarks, or we might be bald, or have flat feet or bad vision, one of our legs might be longer than the other, or we might not be perfectly symmetrical. Is this to say we will always have these weaknesses? No, neither will people live through eternity not knowing what gender they are. This isn't to judge these people who struggle with their sexuality; it is a weakness, just like maintaining healthy body fat is much harder for some than it is for others. But our weaknesses can be made our strengths, either in this life or the next, through our humility and faith.[400] This does not go along with the thought, "I was born this way and there is nothing I can do about it." We must each realize our potential as sons and daughters of God, take responsibility for our own lives, and be all that we can be. Then have hope and faith that in the next life everything will be made right, because it will.

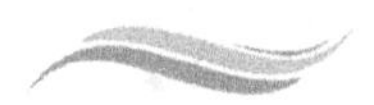

A deeper understanding and appreciation of who we are, and whose we are, prepares us to experience peace within. This understanding and peace helps to alleviate the ill effects of stress. If we come to understand we each have unlimited potential and individual worth, not because of what we do in life (our achievements or how much we accumulate), but rather just because we are a son or daughter of God, and have been given the gift of life, then all our achievements in life will take on a whole new meaning. We won't see our accomplishments as a way to gain our self-esteem, or feelings of importance, but rather a way to serve God and our fellow man.

As mentioned in the mind section, the term self-esteem is used often in our society, but a better word might be *individual worth*. Our individual worth is something we are born with.[401] Our life is a gift from God, not something we acquired through our own beauty, talents, or individual accomplishments. If we really internalize this and apply this principle to our lives, we likely will not put so much pressure on ourselves, and we will be filled with love for God and our fellow man, and a desire to serve them. Wouldn't this be a much better motivating force than fear that if we don't do this or that our self-esteem will suffer?

If we trust God and His plan for us the daily troubles and tribulations of life will take on more of an eternal perspective. Worldly attitudes and pressures won't rob us of our peace and resulting good health. If we lose a loved one to death, we will know that we will see them in the next life. The time of separation will still be hard and reason for mourning, but the faith of life after death will cause us to celebrate the life of the loved one and nurture the hope that we will soon be together again.

QUESTION EVERYTHING?
HEY GRANDMA, HOW COME YOU LOVE ME SO MUCH?
QETommy.com

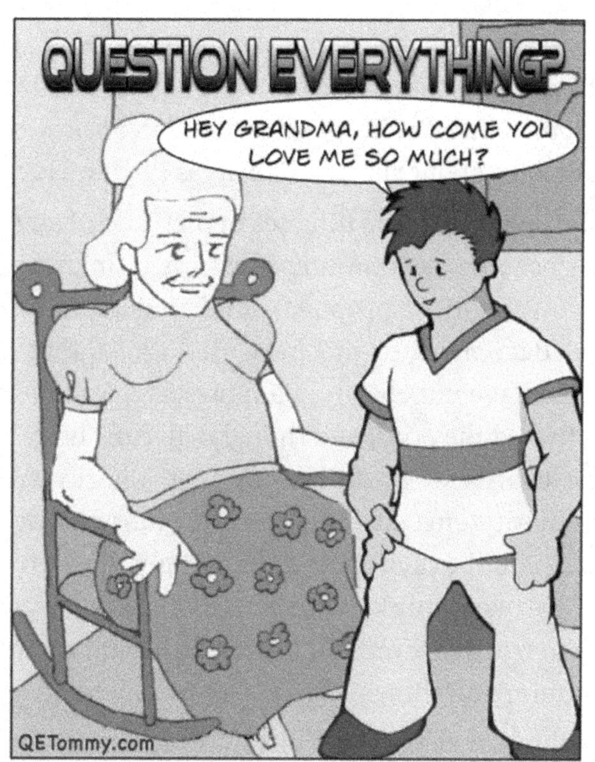

PRINCIPLE #3
Love
The great commandment

What is the greatest or most important commandment?

"Then one of them, which was a lawyer, asked him a question, tempting him, and saying, 'Master, which is the great commandment in the law?' Jesus said unto him, 'Thou shalt love the Lord thy God with all thy heart, and with all thy soul, and with all thy mind. This is the first and great commandment. And the second is like unto it, Thou shalt love thy neighbor as thyself. On these two commandments hang all the law and the prophets."

—Matt. 22: 35-40

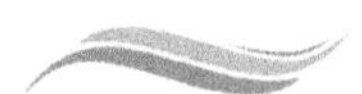

That about sums it up; and this implies we should *love ourselves*. We should see others and ourselves as begotten sons and daughters of God and treat each other as such – we should *love*. One of the most beautiful scriptures in all of holy writ is found in 1 Corinthians Chapter 13, where Paul talks about charity. Charity is the pure love of Christ.[402]

"Though I speak with the tongues of men and of angels, and have not charity, I become as sounding brass, or a tinkling cymbal. And though I have the gift of prophecy, and understand all mysteries, and all knowledge; and though I have all faith, so that I could move mountains, and have not charity, I am nothing. And though I bestow all my goods to feed the poor, and though I give my body to be burned, and have not charity, it profit me nothing. Charity suffereth long, and is kind; charity envyeth not; charity vaunteth not itself, is not puffed up. Doth not behave itself unseemingly, seeketh not her own, is not easily provoked, thinketh no evil. Rejoiceth not in iniquity, but rejoiceth in the truth; beareth all things, believeth all things, hopeth all things, endureth all things. Charity never faileth…"[403]

We may think of charity as a gift to those less fortunate during a special time of the year, or a check written to an institution for those in need. But, best defined, charity is that pure love exemplified by Jesus Christ, and it is a gift of God to all those who search and pray for it, and are true followers of Christ; regardless of whether they believe in Him or not.[404] This gift is not like the worldly love we hear about every day in the media…yes, there may be some truth to the love we hear about, but there are so many lies.

The world would have us believe that we have no control over love. We cannot control when we love, to whom we love, and if we fall out of love. Much of the love we hear about is more along the lines of physical attraction, which is a good thing, or lust, which is a bad thing.

To say we have no control over this love justifies broken relationships and skipping from one partner to another trying to find

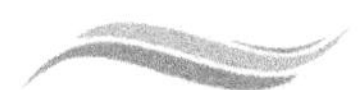

"true love." Yes, physical attraction is important. One of the purposes of this book is to help people be more physically attractive to their spouse, or their future spouse, but there is so much more. If we depend upon lust to fulfill the physical desires we have been blessed with, good luck, it will never happen. We must bridle our passions to be filled with love.[405]

This does not mean it is evil or wrong to feel the amazing emotions and feelings that are associated with physical attraction, or to have wonderful sexual experiences with our spouse; they are good and a gift from God. But true love, charity, is only given to the righteous, those who seek after it, pray for it, and live true to the principles which govern it.[406]

"The greater a man's soul, the deeper he loves."

—Leonardo Da Vinci

If you are fortunate enough to be with a spouse right now who you bond with BodyMindSpirit, one you feel true charity for, and they for you, you are most fortunate indeed. It is not by accident. You are doing something right. This doesn't mean you have sinned if you haven't found it yet. Your time just hasn't come; it will if you live true to it. If you are married to someone who is not there with you, or you are not there with them, in any or all of the most important areas... you can change, and so can they, but there must be a sincere desire and commitment on both your parts to make the relationship work and make the necessary changes.

Go rent the movie, *Fireproof.* It is a glorious movie about a husband and wife that were on the verge of divorce, but through a lot of hard work, prayer, and faith, they allow God to change them and their relationship. Why would anyone not want these sweetest of all the feelings of life? Maybe because they do not know where to find them? If they did, they would have to be crazy to not do everything in their power to get them. There are crazy people out there (we are all

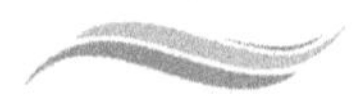

a little crazy), and some are crazier than others... remember all of us must be under the spell of temporary insanity when we live contrary to God's commandments.[407] If we are blessed with God's love in great abundance, we will be selfless with our spouse and with others.

What about those who have gone over the edge, those who are caught up in the pleasures of the world? Does God love the righteous person more than the wicked person? He loves us all equally. He is not a respecter of persons (see Acts 10:34), for all are alike unto God. (See Romans 10:12) The Savior said in Revelations 3:20, "Behold I stand at the door and knock: if *any* man hear my voice, and open the door, I will come in to him, and will sup with him, and he with me." God's love and blessings are available to us *all*, if we chose to allow them into our lives. God favors the righteous with blessings, but He loves us all the same.

How does all this relate to us individually?

"If you judge people, you have no time to love them."

—Mother Teresa

Does this mean we shouldn't judge one another? Maybe what Mother Teresa is saying here is to stop spending so much time gossiping and making final judgments about people, and love them?

"Judge not that ye be not judged."

—Matt. 7:1

We have to make judgments every day about people. Should I walk down that alley? Should I go on a date with this person? Should I trust my child with this responsibility? We have to make judgments every day. We just need to make sure they are *righteous* judgments, and we must not make final judgments.

How about the sinner, how should we feel about them? First of all, "he that is without sin among you, let him first cast a stone." (John

8:7) We need to learn to hate the sin but love the sinner, especially ourselves. This is a hard thing to do sometimes, especially if the sinner has caused us a lot of pain for their sinful acts. How does it feel to be sexually abused by a family member or neighbor, and carry these scars for years? Fortunately, many of us will never know these feelings. Sometimes forgiveness is a very hard thing to do. How does Heavenly Father feel when we sin and live contrary to His plan of happiness? How did He feel when He saw his sinless Son sacrificed for the sins of the world? God understands. Turn to Him, and He will heal you!

"Love is the very essence of life...it is the security for which children weep...it is service to others with no apparent recompense for ourselves...it is the force that can erase the differences between people and bridge the chasms of bitterness...it is the basic essence of goodness...it is the most powerful and enduring virtue...it is probably the most difficult commandment to live but it has the greatest effect upon our lives and those around us...He who most beautifully taught this everlasting truth was the Son of God...In the ultimate expression of love, He did something for us that we could not do for ourselves"

—Gordon B. Hinckley

"For God so loved the world that he gave his only begotten Son, that whosoever believeth in him should not perish, but have everlasting life. For God sent not his Son to condemn the world; but that the world through him might be saved."

—John 3:16, 17

What effect will the love of God and our fellowmen have upon our lives? The blessings are unbelievable...the greatest being eternal life. We will have the opportunity to grow and progress and become like our Heavenly Father.[408] We will follow the Savior with a pure heart and clean hands. We will avoid the pitfalls of pride and not get caught up in the sins of the world and all the suffering that is associated with them. We will have deep and meaningful relationships with our spouse, family members, friends, and associates, and be satisfied and fulfilled to the greatest possible degree. We will not contend one with another. We will be forgiven, for "charity shall cover the multitude of sins." (1 Peter 4:8) We will develop our talents and be an influence for good because the Lord will choose to place us in positions of important leadership where we can set a good example and bring the Gospel to light. We will have great joy, self-esteem (individual worth), and be truly happy. Is there any wonder why charity is the greatest of all?

God loves us perfectly. He will never disappoint us or let us down. Let us turn to Him, so we may feel His love, which is charity, and be blessed with this love, and thus be better able to love God, ourselves, and our fellowmen.

There is a true story about a guy that jumped out of an airplane at 10,000 feet and his parachute didn't open.[409] He hit the ground at full speed and lived to talk about it, amazing. He looks as good as new but told of his *years* in the hospital recovering. He broke almost every bone in his body. He actually died for 20 some minutes on the operating table then came back to life. He talked about his experience and the tunnel of light we often hear about. He said he then met the Savior and that the Savior was interested in two main things:

1. Did he love?

2. Did he receive love?

He was then told that he would be healed, so he could tell of this experience to others and help them to understand that there is life after death, and what is most important in life. He also said it was really hard to leave that place he was in because of the love he felt there. It was comparable to nothing he had ever felt before. Maybe his experience will strengthen your faith in an afterlife and what's most important? Deep down most of us know what he's saying is true, but sometimes it is good to hear true stories like this to strengthen our faith. This man died, but he still continued to live through his spirit.

QUESTION EVERYTHING?
MOM, IF A PICTURE IS WORTH A THOUSAND WORDS, HOW MUCH IS A GOOD EXAMPLE WORTH?
QETommy.com

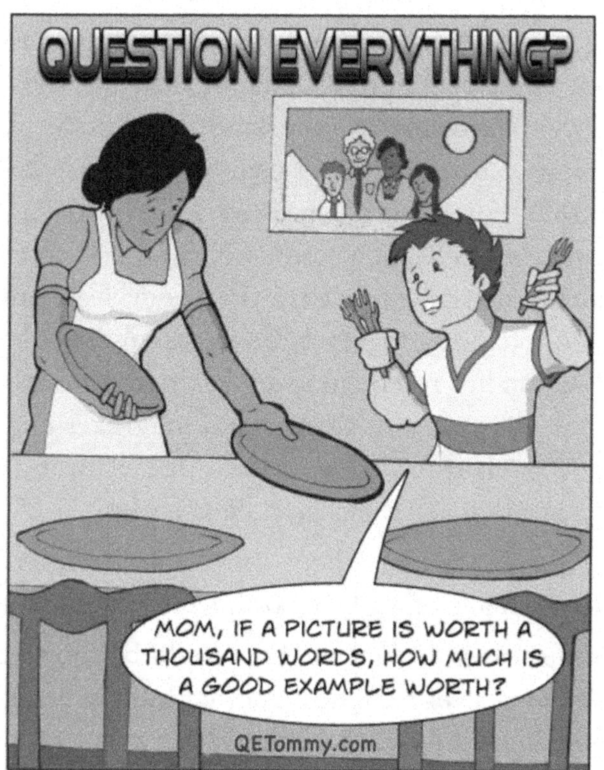

PRINCIPLE #4
Keep Yourself Clean
Have a pure heart and clean hands

"There is no real excellence in all this world which can be separated from right living."

—David Starr Jordan

This is why pornography is so very evil. Avoid it like the plague. It is very addictive, and it will destroy you and your family relationships. If you want to spice things up, become healthier, BodyMindSpirit.

Pray for charity. Pray for a fun, fulfilling relationship with your spouse. Live true to the principles that govern great relationships. Get your body in shape. Eat right, exercise, lose the body fat, tone up your muscles; get the testosterone, estrogen, and endorphins flowing. Keep the romance alive. Or get it back into your relationship. Get out and do something fun. Take a trip. Have a weekly date. Take a stroll along a moonlit beach. Rent a convertible and take a drive, up US 1 or the Pacific Coast Highway (PCH). Go to a drive-in movie. Share a good book. Go to church together. Go shopping together. Buy her a rose. Send him a note. Tell them you love them. Show them you love them. Listen to your partner. Understand their likes and dislikes. Be there for them. Nurture them and encourage them to develop their talents. Lift a burden. Tell them they are beautiful.

Sincerely compliment them...these are the things great relationships are made of. Not the sordid and corrupting influences.

Marriage is a wonderful thing. It should be the most satisfying relationship we will ever have with another human being. We should do everything in our power to ensure this relationship is one of respect, love, fulfillment, happiness, joy, and satisfaction, all within God's commandments. This is where God would have us find our greatest joy.

In 1996, there were 7,874,000 fatherless families with children under the age of 18 years in the U.S. In the same year 1,260,000 children, or 32% of all live births, were born to single mothers.[410] Hollywood increasingly portrays premarital sex as normal and rarely shows the consequences of these acts. But the reality is they are helping to destroy millions of people lives. How many thousands of children went to bed crying last night because of instability at home? Do we really understand the consequences of our actions, or our lack of action? What are we doing to our most prized possessions, our children? We must teach our children the consequences of sin and set a good example for them.

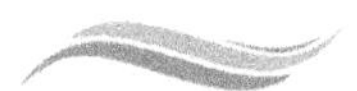

If we have a child who has gone astray, it will hurt, but we must love them and hope that they will come back. We may take comfort in the scripture:

"Train up a child in the way he should go: and when he is old, he will not depart from it."

—Proverbs 22:6

God's only sorrow is for the sins of the world[411]... if we lived a perfect life, which none of us will, this is the only sorrow we would feel, sorrow for others' sins.

"Many sorrows shall be to the wicked: but he that trusteth in the Lord, mercy shall compass him about."

—Psalms 32:10

Despair comes because of iniquity.[412] It is right to feel sorrow for our sins, the sins of our children, our spouse, or the world, but if we are in despair, we need to make some changes. If we are feeling alone, unloved, unappreciated, like nothing we do matters; we are probably doing something wrong. We should evaluate our lives, and put our hearts, minds and souls back into the scriptures, and prayer, and recognize God loves us, we are His children, and we have unlimited potential.

"Be in subjection unto the father of our spirits, and live."

—Heb 12:9

We should "hopeth all things, endureth all things" —1 Cor. 13, and keep God's commandments. Then and only then will we overcome our despair and sorrows and truly be happy.

We are in the Last Days before the Second Coming of the Son of God.[413] It is a time prophesied from the beginning of the world to be very corrupt, some of the worst of times the world has ever known. But it is also a time when the works of righteousness will abound;

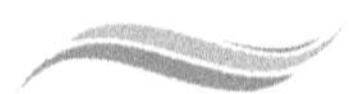

the greatest age the world has ever known. Take a look at what we have been able to accomplish in the last 200 years, it is truly amazing when you look at the history of the world as a whole. This balance of the best of times and the worst of times has to exist. Remember the analogy of the coin? We as a nation and world have increasingly neglected and strayed from time-honored virtues that have shaped our world, proven principles established over centuries of time that are right and good and true.

"You used the name of Deity in the Declaration of Independence and in the Constitution of the United States, yet you cannot use it in the classroom?" (Former Prime Minister of Great Britain, Margaret Thatcher) The voices of a select few are taking precedence over the voices of the masses. We are neglecting God, our Father who made us. America was founded on a belief in God. The Constitution was inspired of God, and it was designed for a righteous people and will not work for any other.[414] *"Our Constitution was made only for a moral and religious people. It is wholly inadequate to the government of any other."*

—John Adams

Righteousness should be the focus in our world, to fix our problems by creating a more righteous and moral people; not by force, but through example, and teaching true and correct principles.

"The American Constitution is, so far as I can see, the most wonderful work ever struck off at a given time by the brain and purpose of man."

—William Gladstone

If the founders of the Constitution saw our world today and some of the things that are allowed in the form of "free speech," they would turn over in their graves.

Between 1972 and 1990, there were 27 million abortions performed in the United States.[415] Up until 2003 when President

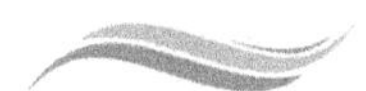

Bush signed a ban on partial birth abortions, we were practicing partial birth abortions; where the baby is turned in the womb and delivered feet first, but before the head of the baby is pulled out, the baby is killed by sucking out its brains. Then their body parts were sold for tens of thousands of dollars.[416] What are we doing? Abortion may be justified in certain situations, like rape and incest, but to be killing babies? The Lord cannot look upon sin with the least degree of allowance.[417] We are allowing the condemnation of God to come upon us because of our wickedness.

Currently America has more than 2 *million* people in prison.[418] We cannot build prisons fast enough to accommodate the need. Gangs, violence, drug abuse and broken homes are sweeping through our nation. What are we doing to ourselves and families? We need people who will stand up and be counted. We need YOU to raise your voice for everything that is good and right and true, and thus confront everything that is evil, wicked and destructive.

If we do nothing, things will only get worse.

Many of the leaders in today's world do not believe their private lives have anything to do with their public office, or their public responsibilities. Please do not become a leader like this. If you have been this way, stop. Most often those who live lives of private immorality cannot make good moral decisions for us in public office or cannot set a good example for our children who look up to them because they are in the limelight. If God cannot trust them, how can we trust them? That is not to say we should not look at the issues and where a politician or leader stands, or if they are corrupt that they cannot make good decisions, because they can, but many use their power and positions for financial or sexual favors, or just have a lust for more power, money, or praise, with no real consideration for those they serve. They place their own selfish desires ahead of the greater good of mankind. This is one of the major reasons things get so out of balance in America's free society. Politicians, corporate

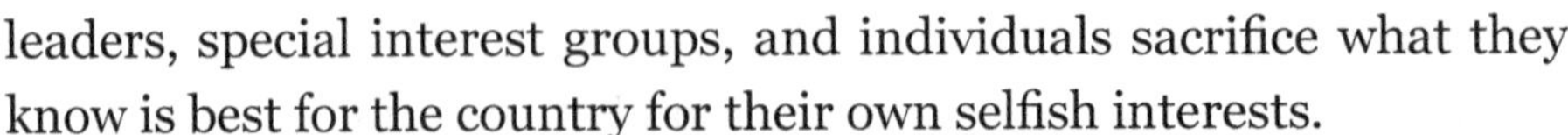

leaders, special interest groups, and individuals sacrifice what they know is best for the country for their own selfish interests.

Many professional athletes, musicians, and actors say they have no responsibility to be a good example to our youth, but the reality is they do have a responsibility, because millions of kids look up to them and copy their every move. We as parents have the great responsibility to be good leaders and teach our children the difference between right and wrong, so corrupt people and negative influences do not sway our youth and lead them down a path of mediocrity and destruction.

How blessed are those children who are brought up in the ways of the Lord from their youth.[419] It makes life so much easier if we are taught from our youth to avoid many of the learning curves that are set in all our paths to help us return to God. Nobody can escape the trials of life, but the rougher the edges, the harder it is to round those edges out, and somehow, we are always given trials that are specific to the things we need to learn in life to progress and one day become perfect.[420] Nobody can escape the trials of life, but we can make life a whole lot easier. Some trials are just part of life, but others come into our lives because of sin.[421] We do have freedom to choose, but we must accept the consequences of our actions. Why make life any harder than it has to be?

If we want to be good, and the good life is the easiest and best way to live, then why be just a little good? Why not be as good as we can be? Kind of like the Army saying, "Be all that you can be." The Lord does not like fence sitters. He says so in the scriptures,

"I know thy works, that thou art neither cold nor hot: I would thou wert cold or hot. So then because thou art lukewarm, and neither cold nor hot, I will spew thee out of my mouth."

—Revelation 3:15, 16

It doesn't do any good to pout with the Lord and become a fence sitter because things aren't going the way we think they should...we

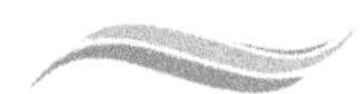

just have to accept life as it comes, hope the Lord knows what He's doing (which He does), and move forward with faith. This means, be as good as we can be. Live a life of "*No Regrets.*"

How will we feel if we miss living with God through time and eternity, if we miss the goal of eternal life and eternal progression, by dropping out at the last moment? How will we feel? The sad reality is many people will. Some people live a life of greatness then give up at the last moment. Or they give up somewhere along the way when they are tried and tested. We must *endure to the end* to win the prize.[422] One of the most remembered speeches Winston Churchill ever gave was also his shortest. He was expected to give a great long speech about an interesting topic but instead stood up and said the following: "*Never, never, never give up.*"[423] Then he sat down. What a great lesson about enduring to the end.

There's a great line from the movie *Field of Dreams*, where the main character's (Kevin Costner) father is asking him if he is in heaven. Kevin says, "No, this is Iowa." Then his father says, "It sure feels like heaven," and Kevin replies, "Maybe it is." Then one of them says, "Heaven is a place where all your dreams come true." If there is anything that has caused you true joy and happiness in this life, if you are true and faithful you will have it in the world to come. If there is anything you didn't accomplish in this life, you can do it in the next. Let's play fill-in-the-blank:

Will there be ________________________ (your favorite) in heaven? Yes!

But in order to achieve these things in the next life, and have peace and joy in this life, we must come to God and stay there. If we wander, we must speedily repent and come back to the Lord's side. There will be no fence sitters in heaven. It's OK if you fall off the straight and narrow path, we all do, just make sure you cross the straight and narrow as much as possible.

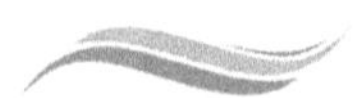

Why do so many blessings in life come *after* the trial of our faith? Do you notice this too? Maybe the Lord is seeing how much we really desire the blessings we seek? He wants to see if we will bow out at the last moment; if we will doubt ourselves, the Lord, His word, His grace? The Lord stands at the door and knocks; will we let Him in?[424]

If we fail in life, or at the things we do in life, it's not because the Lord didn't do His part, it will be because we didn't do ours. We tried to do it on our own without His help and it didn't work. How sad.

"Of all the words of tongue and pen, the saddest are these – it might have been."

—John Whittier

Don't let this be your lot in life. Live a life of *No Regrets.* Stay close to God, for He truly will make a whole lot more out your life than you can. If you have made mistakes, join the crowd. Repent. All is not lost. You might have missed out on some wonderful blessings; but you can still achieve the most important blessing, eternal life with God. Don't beat yourself up or live in the past, move forward and live life in the present. If God has forgiven you, forgive yourself. Life is wonderful, you are greater than you could ever imagine.

There is a great saying that has a double meaning. It is a combination of a couple inspiring quotes, it says, DOn't quIT NOW. A saying by Nike says, Just Do It, which, propels us to action. One of our world's great men, Spencer W. Kimball, had the saying on his desk, Do It Now, which calls us to immediate action. If we have been faithful, we must not falter. We must come to God and endure to the end, Don't Quit Now. Thus, to combine all three of these sayings we get the saying, DOn't quIT NOW. Maybe these simple sayings will help you? Or find your own that inspire you and put them out where you see them every day.

QUESTION EVERYTHING?
ANASTASIA, WILL YOU BE MY GIRLFRIEND?
QETommy.com

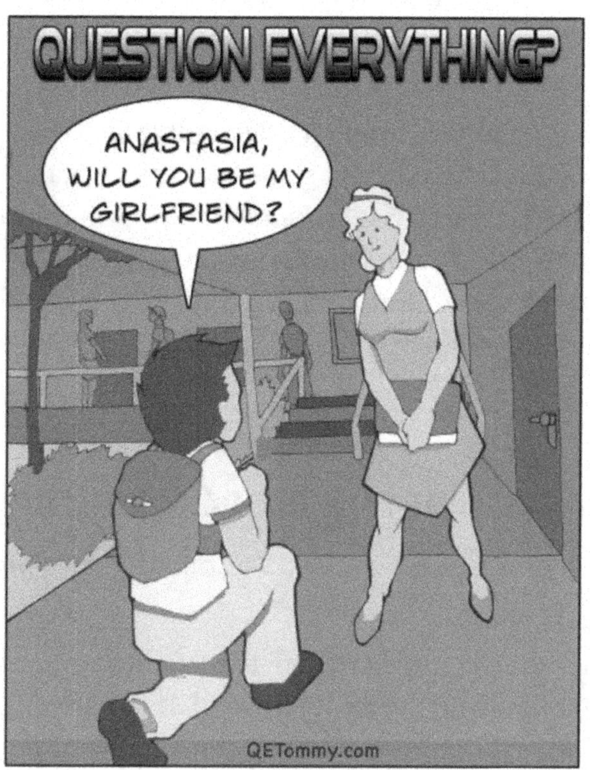

PRINCIPLE #5
Focus On Your Family

They will be your greatest source of joy

Our greatest calling in life will be to be a good husband, wife, son, or daughter.

"The most important work you will ever do will be within the walls of your own home."

—David O. McKay

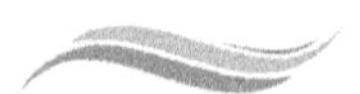

Our greatest joys in life will come from our family. The family is also where our greatest sorrows in life can be. It will be what we and our family members make of it.

There is a great talk from an outstanding man named David O. McKay. It is a direct and correct statement that explains our purpose here on earth.[425] It is a Christian belief that we will be accountable to Christ after this life, we will be asked about our works here on earth. If you cannot picture Christ asking you these things, picture God, a Higher Power, or a parent or grandparent asking you this after you die:

ACCOUNT FOR RESPONSIBILITIES

(Written to men but just as applicable to women)

"Let me assure you brethren that someday you will have a personal interview with the Savior himself. If you are interested, I will tell you the *order* in which he will ask you to account for your earthly responsibilities.

FIRST: He will request an accountability report about your relationship with your wife. Have you been actively engaged in making her happy and ensuring that her needs have been met as an individual?

SECOND: He will want an accountability report about each of your children, individually. He will not attempt to have this for simply a family stewardship but will request information about your relationship to each and every child.

THIRD: He will want to know what you have personally done with the talents you have been given...

FOURTH: He will want a summary of your activity in your Church assignments. He will not necessarily be interested in

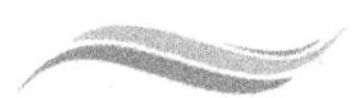

what assignments you had...but He will request a summary of how you have been of service to your fellowmen in your Church assignments.

FIFTH: He will have no interest in how you earned your living, but if you were honest in all your business dealings.

SIXTH: He will ask for an accountability on what you have done to contribute in a positive manner to your community, state, country, and the world."

Our first and most important responsibilities are to our spouse and children. If you desire true joy in life, you will focus your efforts first on your spouse, then on your children, making sure their needs are met. Man's role is that of a husband, father, provider, and protector. Woman's role is that of a wife, mother, nurturer, and helpmate to her husband. This might sound very old fashioned and not realistic in today's world, but we, male and female, are very different. Each are of equal worth and value, neither the man nor the woman is above the other. But we each have very special and specific talents and abilities. We can do things our spouse cannot do, or at least not as good.

Women have a unique love that comes from God; they can love in ways known only to God, maybe it is their mothering instinct? Women are very special before the Lord. They are to be loved and protected. They possess great charity which is the "greatest of all the gifts of God."

Men have tremendous strength, physically and in other ways. From the first man, Adam, men were commanded to be the protector and provider. This is not to say women cannot do a better job at providing, because many times they can, but their greatest gifts are more needed with the children.

"The hand that rocks the cradle is the hand that rules the world."

—William Ross Wallace

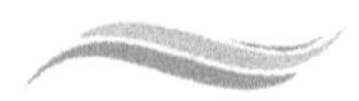

Children are our greatest natural resource. They are more important than wealth, our careers, or the conveniences of life.

Many children in today's world spend more time with babysitters than they do with their own parents. It is sad to note all the children who come home to an empty home these days. 30 years ago, the number children left at home without adequate supervision was one million.[426] Today that number has doubled to two million.[427]

"There is no way of measuring the emotional damage suffered by inadequately supervised children or the later costs of delinquency which results from this failure."

—Gertrude Hoffman – U.S. Children's Bureau

Let's talk a bit about developing our great talents and abilities we are blessed with, as it will be one of the questions the Savior asks us in our interview with Him. We each have them in different areas and in different amounts. Do you remember the parable of the talents in the scriptures? (Matt. 25:14-30) A man had three servants, to one he gave one talent, to another he gave two, and the other he gave five, each according to their several abilities. The servants with the two and five talents went to the exchangers and doubled their talents, but the servant with one talent buried his in the sand and did not earn any more. After a long time, the lord came to his servants and asked them what they had done with their talents. To the two who developed their talents into more he said:

"Well done thou good and faithful servant: thou hast been faithful over a few things, I will make thee ruler over many things: enter thou into the joy of thy lord." When the lord asked the servant with one talent what he had done with his he gave this response: "Lord, I knew thee that thou art an hard man, reaping where thou hast not sown, and gathering where thou hast not strawed: And I was afraid, and I went and hid thy talent in the earth: lo, there thou hast that is thine."

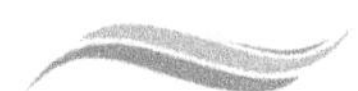

To which his lord answered, "Thou wicked and slothful servant, thou knewest that I reap where I sowed not, and gather where I have not strawed: Thou oughtest therefore to have put my money to the exchangers, and then at my coming I should have received mine own with usury. Take therefore the talent from him, and give unto him which hath ten talents. For unto every one that hath shall be given, and he shall have in abundance: but from him that hath not shall be taken away even that which he hath. And cast ye the unprofitable servant into outer darkness: there shall be weeping and gnashing of teeth."

—Matt. 25:14-30

This might seem cruel, but we cannot let fear stop us from developing the great talents each of us are blessed with. It doesn't matter how many talents we have; we just need to develop them. Don't bury them in the sand! As a father you might be a great athlete; you have the ability to set a good example for your family of being fit, and an athlete, showing your kids the in's and out's of sport and how they can develop their great talents and be healthy through exercise and sport. As a mother you might have a great gift for music; you can fill your home and family's life with beautiful music and inspire your children to develop their musical talents and do the same for their families the rest of their lives. Or you might be a single person that is a wiz with the computer; you might have the ability to start your own computer company, make lots of money, and help many people. Whatever your talents are develop them. We are under sacred responsibility to do all we can to bless other's lives with the great gifts and talents we've been given.

Remember what is most important in life and keep things in balance.

It will be really sad to stand in front of the Savior when he asks you, "Where is your family?"

And you have nothing to say other than, "Well, I was too busy doing this or that, or I met this person when I was married, or, I didn't love them anymore" ...these excuses will be very hollow before the Lord.

Many people develop their talents to glorify themselves, to make themselves feel important. Some people achieve much success and attribute it to their own wisdom, hard work and talent. Where did they get that talent? Where did they acquire that knowledge? Who really owns all that we possess? God is the giver of life; everything we have is Gods.[428] In the great movie, *Chariots of Fire*, when a friend was trying to get Eric Little to compete on the Sabbath Day and sited a King's approval to compete, Eric said, "God makes Kings."[429] God made us who we are; we should give the credit to Him. If there is anything good in us it is a direct reflection of Him, not us. Yes, we are putting forth the effort, but if we look to God in all we do it is Him who strengthens us and helps us to do things we could never do on our own.

QUESTION EVERYTHING?
GRANDMA, HOW COME SOME PEOPLE GO HUNGRY?
QETommy.com

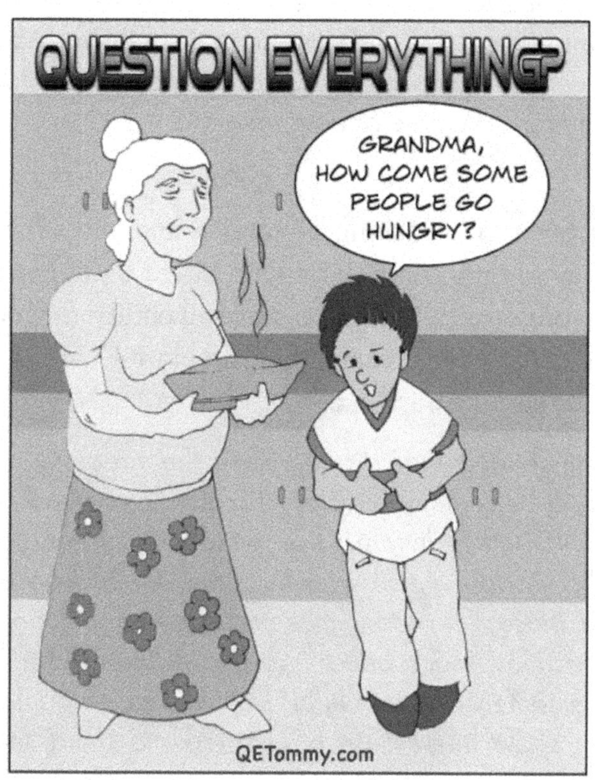

PRINCIPLE # 6
Serve Others

You will only be in the service of our God

Service is an important part of a productive life, as the Savior so lovingly demonstrated.

"For I was an hungered, and ye gave me meat: I was thirsty, and ye gave me drink: I was sick, and ye visited me: I was in prison, and ye came unto me. Then shall the righteous answer him, saying, Lord when saw we thee an hungered, and fed thee? Or thirsty, and gave thee drink? When saw we thee a stranger, and took thee in? Or

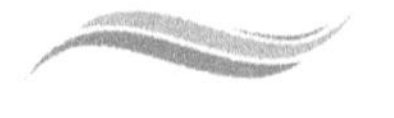

naked, and clothed thee? Or when saw we thee sick, or in prison, and came unto thee? And the King shall answer and say unto them, Verily I say unto you, inasmuch as ye have done it unto the least of these my brethren, ye have done it unto me."

—Matt. 25:35-40

What a beautiful teaching of service and the worth of a soul. God didn't say to only serve those who might be of benefit to us, or only those in our family. We are to serve all children of our Heavenly Father; for when we serve each other, no matter who they might be, we will only be serving our God.[430]

"Service is the virtue that distinguishes the great of all times and which they will be remembered by. It places a mark of nobility upon its disciples. It is the dividing line which separates the two great groups of the world – those who help and those who hinder, those who lift and those who lean, those who contribute and those who only consume. How much better it is to give than to receive. Service in any form is comely and beautiful. To give encouragement, to impart sympathy, to show interest, to banish fear, to build self-confidence and awaken hope in the hearts of others – in short, to love them and to show it – is to render the most precious service."

—Stephen Covey

Is some service better than another? The purest forms of service are those where we do something for others that they cannot do for themselves[431]; maybe serving those who have handicaps, those who are children, the aged, those who are hungry, those with no good clothing, etc. How about those who are beggars and could actually get a job if they really wanted to? If people ask, we should help.[432] It's not easy to discern true need.

In New York City, and most every city in the world, every single day people ask others for money...it's so very sad. Some people will take money without even a thank you. But others are so appreciative

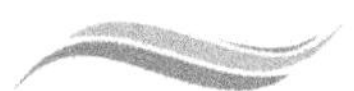

you can hardly believe it. Some people will be on the streets crying. Sometimes you wonder if they are just putting on a show or if they really are that desperate. It is not for us to judge, for are we not all beggars? Do we not all depend upon the same being, even God, for all that we have and are, even our daily breath and bread?[433]

"Freely ye have received, freely give."

—Matt. 10:8

Should we let people put their petitions up to us in vain? Does God do the same for us? If we served God all the day long, if we rendered all the thanks and praise that our whole bodies possessed, yet we would be unprofitable servants. For God grants unto us our very lives, He created us from the beginning, He preserves us from day to day, lending us breath; that we may live and move according to the dictates of our own conscience, supporting us from one moment to the other.[434] Why do we forget this? Why are we so ungrateful in our prayers and the desires of our hearts?

Remember the ten lepers in the scriptures that were cleansed and only one returned to thank the Lord?[435] Are we like the one that came back to thank the Lord, or like the other nine? Are we like those beggars who don't even say thanks for the handout? Or the others that are truly thankful? If you were Heavenly Father, which one of these people would you rather help? Or which one would you more likely give an eternal reward? Should we let any of these people put up their petitions to us in vain? Why do we allow anyone to go hungry or live on the streets? It's not God's fault; it's our fault.

"Give to him that asketh thee, and from him that would borrow of thee turn not away"

—Matt. 5:42

The earth has more than enough.[436] It is because of the greediness and gluttony of man that others go hungry. Our earth's resources are

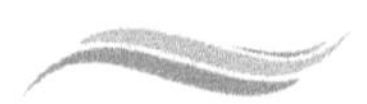

plentiful; there is more than enough and to spare. God is good and kind and loving. He doesn't want people to go hungry. He doesn't want people living in the streets with no place to sleep. Why do we mess it all up?

It is touching to read about people that give money and goods away to help the less fortunate, it's even more touching to read about the less fortunate being blessed and nobody knowing who gave it. These are the kinds of people our world needs. Those who make the money, then give it away to help others. This is the very reason God gives these things to us, so we can give them away to help others.[437] The scriptures teach us that if we really desire wealth God will grant it to us, but we must first seek the kingdom of God and His righteousness.

"No servant can serve two masters: for either he will hate the one, and love the other; or else he will hold to the one and despise the other. Ye cannot serve God and mammon."

—Luke 16:13

This is why we should pray with all the energy of heart that we may be filled with this love, and be true followers of God, so He will bestow this love upon us in great abundance.[438]

If you were God, wouldn't you choose individuals who are motivated by this love to help you in your work to bring to pass the immortality and eternal life of man? If we desire to truly serve God, we must possess this love, and if we do God will use us in His work.

QUESTION EVERYTHING?
"MR. PIRATE, DO YOU TAKE FROM THE RICH TO GIVE TO THE POOR?"
QETommy.com

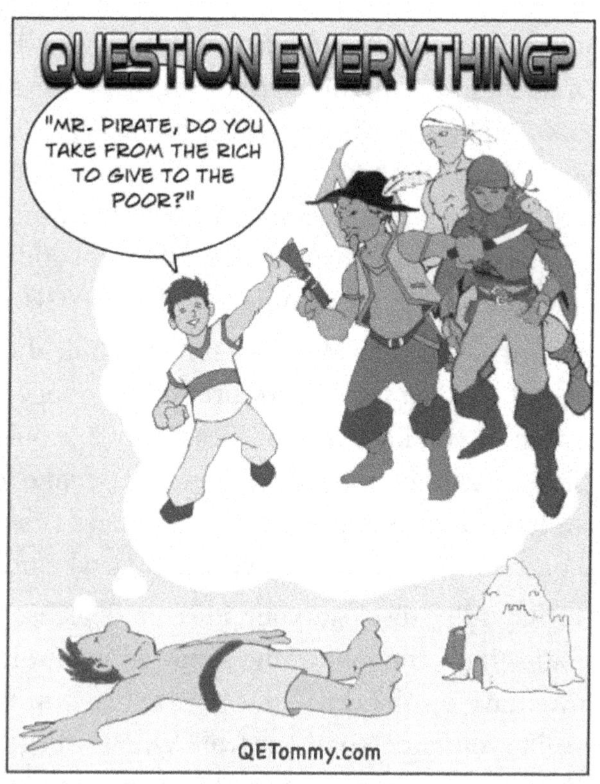

PRINCIPLE # 7
Use a BodyMindSpirit Approach to the Development of Your Spirit
Anything less and you go in circles

The spiritual side of our nature is the most important to develop and focus on. But it will be much easier to develop your spirituality if you are physically fit, and mentally sound. We cannot separate our bodies, minds and spirits; they function together in great harmony. You will create great synergy between them if you have good balance and develop all three areas.

Your time and attention is greatly appreciated, thank you so much for reading this book! As a company family (WAVE) your input is greatly appreciated; you might have some great ideas about how to make the book, TV show, websites, or company better. Please let us know what you think, and how we can better serve you, please feel free to write: QETommy@icloud.com Your greatness and goodness is of great value to us and to God, you are His great son or daughter. You are of unfathomable worth; Heavenly Father loves YOU.

One of the things we do in WAVE is not only talk about the value we see in you, but we also implement programs to incorporate your ideas and wisdom. If you have a great idea that you would like to put into action, please write to us and let us know. To make ideas work it usually takes financial backing and sound business practices. If you would like to partner up with WAVE we might also be interested.

Please do not fully disclose your idea, and please realize that someone else may have thought of the same thing, but if you will fill out the form we have on the wave4life.com website under "Business Ideas", and we like your idea, someone from WAVE will get back to you with a call. We've given much attention to ensuring that this filtering process is as fair as possible, and many people will consider your idea. If people like what you have to say in your form, we will contact you and set up a meeting. Your idea might be the next direction of the company; your idea might change our world.

Thanks again so much for your time and attention. God bless you!

QUESTION EVERYTHING?
PIRATE TAHOE, HAVE YOU TRIED PLAYING FOOTBALL?
QETommy.com

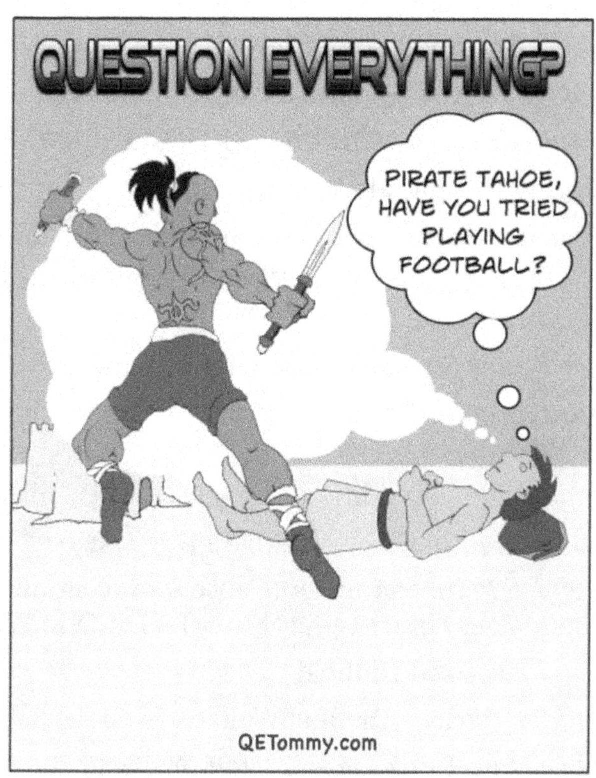

APPENDIX

Suggested Reading Material

Body

1. *The China Study* – Dr. T. Colin Campbell & Thomas M. Campbell II
2. *Eat To Live* – Dr. Joel Fuhrman
3. *Dr. Dean Ornish's Program for Reversing Heart Disease* – Dean Ornish
4. *The Total Health Solution for the 21st Century* – Dr. John and Mary McDougall

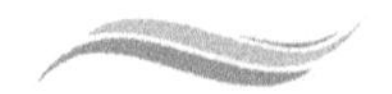

5. *The Pleasure Trap* – Dr. Douglas Lisle
6. *Breaking The Food Seduction* – Dr. Neal Barnard
7. *Original Fast Foods* – Jim & Coleen Simmons
8. *The 80/10/10 Diet* – Dr. Douglas N. Graham
9. *Mega Health* – Dr. Marc Sorenson
10. *The Calcium Factor* – James Barefoot & Dr. Carl Reich
11. *Prevent and Reverse Heart Disease* – Dr. Caldwell B. Esselstyn, Jr.
12. *Bigger Faster Stronger* – Dr. Greg Sheppard
13. *Russian Strength Training Secrets for Every American* – Pavel Tsatsouline
14. *Vitamin Bible* – Earl Mindell
15. *Mind Body Fitness* – Dr. Barbara Day Lockhart
16. *1931 Nobel Prize on Cancer* (Cause & prevention of Cancer; Biochem, Zeits, 152: 514-520, 1924) – Dr. Otto Warburg
17. *Fitness* – Dr. Fred Hatfield
18. *Forbidden Cures* – Dr. Joel Wallach
19. *Dead Doctors Don't Lie* – Dr. Joel Wallach
20. *The Word of Wisdom Today* – Roy Doxey
21. *Fitness for Life* – Phil Alsen
22. *Pumping Iron* – Arnold Schwarzenegger

Mind

1. *The Secret* – various authors
2. *The Road Less Traveled* – Scott Peck
3. *How To Win Friends and Influence People* – Dale Carnegie
4. *Think and Grow Rich* – Napoleon Hill
5. *Mind Over Time* – Doug Warren
6. *Trump: The Art of the Deal* – Donald Trump
7. *The Lessons of History* – Will and Ariel Durant

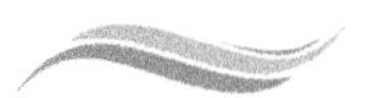

8. *Rich Dad Poor Dad* – Robert Kiyosaki
9. *McDonald's: Behind the Golden Arches* – John Love
10. *As A Man Thinketh* – James Allen
11. *The Hunchback of Notre Dame* – Victor Hugo
12. *Les Misérables* – Victor Hugo
13. *A Farewell to Arms* – Ernest Hemingway
14. *Wealth Without Risk* – Charles Givens
15. *The Age Wave* – Ken Dychtwald
16. *The 7 Habits of Highly Effective People* – Stephen Covey
17. *First Things First* – Stephen Covey
18. *The Classics* – various authors
19. *The Power of Positive Thinking* – Norman Vincent Peale
20. *An Enemy Hath Done This* – Ezra Benson
21. *A Sociological Perspective of Sport* – Wilbert Leonard
22. *The Wellness Industry: How to Make a Fortune in The Next $TRILLION Industry* – Paul Pilzer
23. *The Greatest Salesman in The World* – Og Mandino

Spirit

1. *Jesus The Christ* – James Talmage
2. *The Screwtape Letters* – C.S. Lewis
3. *Mere Christianity* – C.S. Lewis
4. *Pure in Heart* – Dallin Oaks
5. *The Old and New Testament* – God
6. *A Marvelous Work and a Wonder* – LeGrand Richards
7. *You are Greater Than You Know* – Lou Austin
8. *Worth Waiting For* – Brent Barlow
9. *On Wings of Faith* – Fredrick Babbel
10. *Standing For Something* – Gordon B. Hinckley

11. *Be Thou and Example* – Gordon B. Hinckley
12. *Faith: The Essence of True Religion* – Gordon B. Hinckley
13. *The Radiant Life* – Truman Madsen
14. *All These Things Shall Give Thee Experience* – Neal Maxwell
15. *Things As They Really Are* – Neal Maxwell
16. *Why The Religious Life* – Mark Petersen
17. *Enjoy the Journey Along Your Marriage Highway* – Tres & Susan Tanner
18. *The 7 Habits of Highly Effective Families* – Stephen Covey
19. *The Divine Center* – Stephen Covey
20. *Human Intimacy: Illusion & Reality* – Victor Brown
21. *Drawing On the Powers of Heaven* – Grant Von Harrison

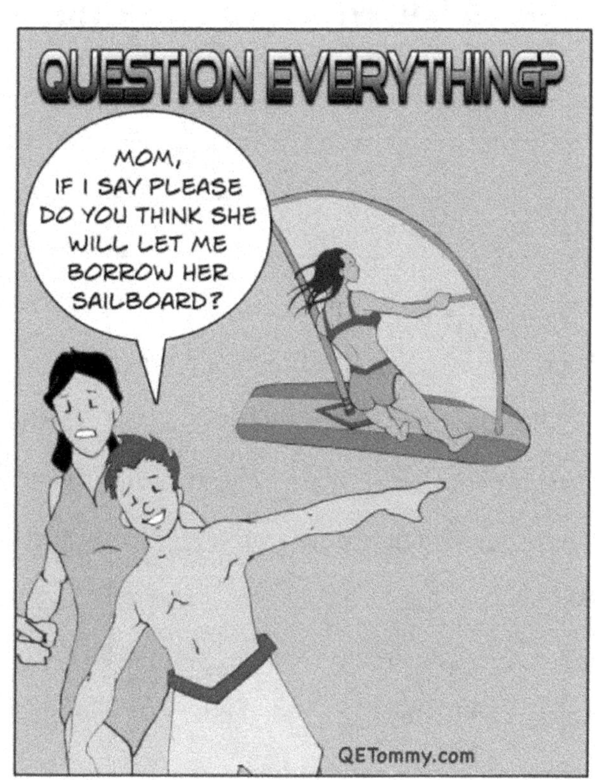
QUESTION EVERYTHING?
MOM, IF I SAY PLEASE DO YOU THINK SHE WILL LET ME BORROW HER SAILBOARD?
QETommy.com

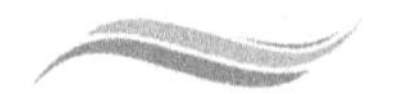

WAVE for Fitness Evaluation

Date: ______________Trainer: ___________________________________

Client Name: ____

Address: ____

Phone:(______) ______________________Cell:(______)

E-Mail Address: _____________________________Birthdate: ________

Resting Heart Rate: ___________Resting Blood Pressure: _____________

Height: _______Weight: ________Body Fat: ________Method: _______

Neck: _____Chest (pecs): ______Arms: _____Waist (belly button): ______

Hips (femur): ________Thighs (largest site): ________Calves: ________

Estimated VO2 Max: ____________________Method: ______________

Sit-Ups (1min.): _______Push-Ups (Max): ________Sit & Reach: ______

Chest Press (10 reps or less): _______Method: ____________1RM: ______

Leg Press (10 reps or less): ______Method: ______________1RM: ______

BRZYCKI EQUATION: 1RM = Wt. Lifted/ 1.0278 - .0279X (X = # of Reps Performed – 10 or less)

Important Note: *When figuring out your 1RM (1 rep max) do not go much below 10 repetitions unless you are used to it! You will injure yourself. Get a weight that you can do about 10 times, then plug that weight into the Brzycki Equation to get your 1RM.*

Norms for your age and gender: After you complete the Fitness Evaluation compare your scores with the YMCA national averages below (see The Y's way to Fitness, 3rd Edition). For other test averages and procedures do a Google search.

PHYSICAL EXAM: It is suggested that you visit your doctor for a complete physical examination before starting any exercise program. It is also good to get your blood work done so you can determine your "inward health" also.

Resting Heart Rate Men

Age	18-25	26-35	36-45	46-55	56-65	66+
Athlete	49-55	49-54	50-56	50-57	51-56	50-55
Excellent	56-61	55-61	57-62	58-63	57-61	56-61
Good	62-65	62-65	63-66	64-67	62-67	62-65
Above Avg	66-69	66-70	67-70	68-71	68-71	66-69
Average	70-73	71-74	71-75	72-76	72-75	70-73
Below Avg	74-81	75-81	76-82	77-83	76-81	74-79
Poor	82+	82+	83+	84+	82+	80+

Resting Heart Rate Women

Age	18-25	26-35	36-45	46-55	56-65	66+
Athlete	54-60	54-59	54-59	54-60	54-59	54-59
Excellent	61-65	60-64	60-64	61-65	60-64	60-64
Good	66-69	65-68	65-69	66-69	65-68	65-68
Above Avg	70-73	69-72	70-73	70-73	69-73	69-72
Average	74-78	73-76	74-78	74-77	74-77	73-76
Below Avg	79-84	77-82	79-84	78-83	78-83	77-84
Poor	85+	83+	85+	84+	84+	84+

1 Minute Sit-Up Test Men

Age	18-25	26-35	36-45	46-55	55-65	66+
Athlete	>49	>45	>41	>35	>31	>28
Excellent	44-49	40-45	35-41	29-35	25-31	22-28
Good	39-43	35-39	30-34	25-28	21-24	19-21
Above Avg	35-38	31-34	27-29	22-24	17-20	15-18
Average	31-34	29-30	23-26	18-21	13-16	11-14
Below Avg	25-30	22-28	17-22	13-17	9-12	7-10
Poor	<25	<22	<17	<9	<9	<7

1 Minute Sit-Up Test Women

Age	18-25	26-35	36-45	46-55	56-65	66+
Athlete	>43	>39	>33	>27	>24	>23
Excellent	37-43	33-39	27-33	22-27	18-24	17-23
Good	33-36	29-32	23-26	18-21	13-17	14-16
Above Avg	29-32	25-28	19-22	14-17	10-12	11-13
Average	25-28	21-24	15-18	10-13	7-9	5-10
Below Avg	18-24	13-20	7-14	5-9	3-6	2-4
Poor	<18	<20	<7	<5	<3	<2

Squat Test Men

Age	18-25	26-35	36-45	46-55	56-65	66+
Excellent	>49	>45	>41	>35	>31	>28
Good	44-49	40-45	35-41	29-35	25-31	22-28
Above Avg	39-43	35-39	30-34	25-38	21-24	19-21
Average	35-38	31-34	27-29	22-24	17-20	15-18
Below avg.	31-34	29-30	23-26	18-21	13-16	11-14
Poor	25-30	22-28	17-22	13-17	9-12	7-10
Very Poor	<25	<22	<17	<9	<9	<7

Squat Test Women

Age	18-25	26-35	36-45	46-55	56-65	66+
Excellent	>43	>39	>33	>27	>24	>23
Good	37-43	33-39	27-33	22-27	18-24	17-23
Above Avg	33-36	29-32	23-26	18-21	13-17	14-16
Average	29-32	25-28	19-22	14-17	10-12	11-13
Below Avg	25-28	21-24	15-18	10-13	7-9	5-10
Poor	18-24	13-20	7-14	5-9	3-6	2-4
Very Poor	<18	<20	<7	<5	<3	<2

Push-Up Test Men

Age	17-19	20-29	30-39	40-49	50-59	60+
Excellent	>56	>47	>41	>34	>31	>30
Good	47-56	39-47	34-41	28-34	25-31	24-30
Above Avg	35-46	30-39	25-33	21-28	18-24	17-23
Average	19-34	17-29	13-24	11-20	9-17	6-16
Below avg.	11-18	10-16	8-12	6-10	5-8	3-5
Poor	4-10	4-9	2-7	1-5	1-4	1-2
Very Poor	<4	<4	<2	0	0	0

Body Fat Test

	general population		athletes	
	males	females	males	females
lean	< 12	< 17	< 7	< 12
acceptable	12 - 17	17 - 23	7 - 13	12 - 20
moderately overweight	18 - 23	24 - 30	14 - 19	21 - 25
overweight	> 24	> 31	>20	>26

Push-Up Test Women

Age	**17-19**	**20-29**	**30-39**	**40-49**	**50-59**	**60+**
Excellent	>35	>36	>37	>31	>25	>23
Good	27-35	30-36	30-37	25-31	21-25	19-23
Above Avg	21-27	23-29	22-30	18-24	15-20	13-18
Average	11-20	12-22	10-21	8-17	7-14	5-12
Below avg.	6-10	7-11	5-9	4-7	3-6	2-4
Poor	2-5	2-6	1-4	1-3	1-2	1
Very Poor	0-1	0-1	0	0	0	0

Sit and Reach Test

	men		**women**	
	cm	**inches**	**cm**	**inches**
Excellent	> +27	> +10	> +30	> +11
Good	+17 to +27	+6 to +10	+21 to +30	+8 to +11
Above Avg	+6 to +16	+2 to +6	+11 to +20	+4 to +7
Average	0 to +5	0 to +2	+1 to +10	0 to +4
Below Avg	-8 to -1	-3 to - 0	-7 to 0	-2 to 0
Poor	-20 to -9	-7 to -3	-15 to -8	-6 to -3
Very Poor	< -20	< -7	< -15	< -6

QUESTION EVERYTHING?
DAD, WHY DO SOME MEN LEAVE THE TOILET SEAT DOWN WHEN THEY PEE?
MEN
QETommy.com

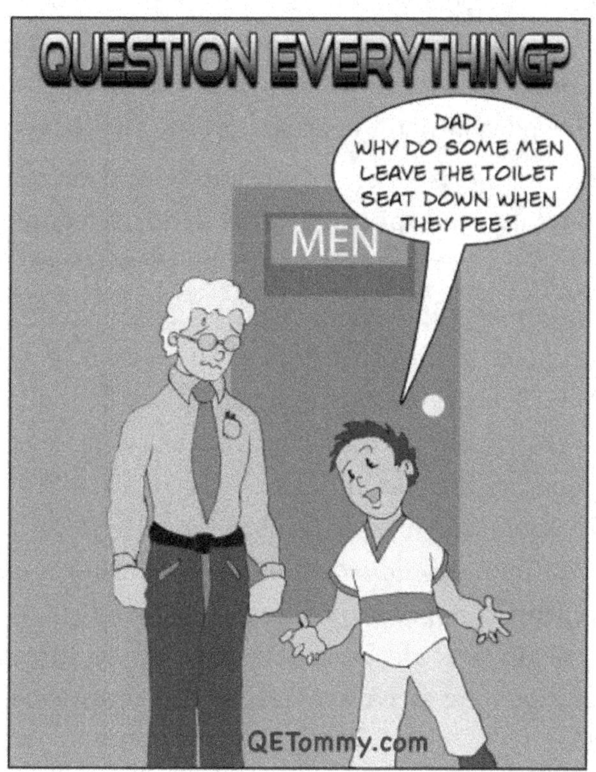

WAVE 4 Fitness 6-Week Challenge

The following is a Challenge in the area of your physical fitness.

If you are young, middle aged, or heading toward your twilight years we would encourage you to adhere to this Challenge for the next 6 weeks of your life, and see if you can significantly improve how you look, feel, and perform your various physical activities.

This Challenge will work for old and young, athlete and inactive, physically fit and obese.

All we're asking is for 15 – 30 minutes a day of your time for the next 6 weeks. Is there anyone out there who cannot do this? Is there anyone out there who shouldn't do this?

If you have ever been an athlete or extremely fit before you know how good it feels. You feel like you can do most anything physically, and your mind and spirit are so much sharper and in tune with your body. If you have never had the great opportunity to feel this, try it.

Your goal in life is likely to be happy and be your best self, physically, mentally, and spiritually. If you are neglecting any of these areas, you are weak. You are only as strong as your weakest link.

We often ignore our physical well-being, or do not achieve our great physical potential because we are so focused on other areas of our lives that we feel are more important. It is true that some aspects of our nature are more important than others, we believe the spiritual aspect of our nature is most important, but it is also true that we are not just spirit, or mind, or body, we are BodyMindSpirit inseparably connected, and thus should work on all three aspects of our nature to provide optimal happiness, balance and synergy. As we become stronger physically, we will become exponentially stronger mentally and spiritually, as long as we are developing all three aspects of our nature together.

What good is it to have a strong mind and spirit but not be able to go about our daily physical activities? Likewise, what good is it to be strong physically, but not have the mental and spiritual strength to live a good life?

If you will take this Challenge to heart and commit only 15 – 30 minutes a day to elevate your physical fitness, you will notice a significant improvement in all aspects of your life. You will also be on the path of setting a great example to those you love the most, your family, of someone who is balanced and happy. Thus, you will be able to help them to do the same, because example is the best teacher.

NOTE: This Challenge is meant to go hand in hand with the Nutritional Analysis, which will help you lose weight (if needed), be full of energy, and enjoy great tasting healthy recipes.

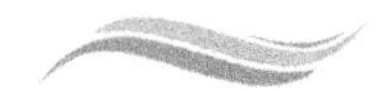

What is the WAVE 4 Fitness Challenge?

WAVE represents **W**orldwide **A**chievement, **V**itality & **E**xcellence. Our goal with this Challenge is to help you achieve more physically and get you into the habit of exercise. This is not a weightlifting program. We have designed a weightlifting program for you if this is your desire, but the most important thing is that you *DO SOMETHING!* It really doesn't matter what it is that you do for your fitness program, as long as it is in line with your fitness objectives. If you don't have a goal figured out yet, get it done. It might take you a couple days to come up with it, you might even need to fast and pray about it, but once you know what it is you want to accomplish then as the Nike saying says, JUST DO IT!

People generally gravitate toward what they are good at. It is much easier to do things that we enjoy. If you are a great basketball player, then set your goal in something to do with basketball...maybe to make 70 out of 100 free throws before the year's end. If you have great natural physical endurance, you might want to run a marathon next year, or join a biking club so you can bike 50 miles in one day this coming summer. Or you might be 90 years old and want to be strong enough to go about your daily activities without the assistance of other people, so your goal is to be able to do 30 squats and 30 push-ups a day by next year. You get the idea. Whatever it is you enjoy and are good at, DO IT!

Our Challenge is for you to work on your goal for at least 15 – 30 minutes a day, 6 days a week, for the next 6 weeks. God himself rested the 7th day so should you. If you cannot do something every day, or miss a day here and there, it is OK, keep going. We have included a chart for you to check off your progress. As you complete a day's work out, check it off. This is very motivating and it will help you complete the Challenge.

The Level 1-3 Programs

We have designed Level 1 – 3 Fitness Programs for you so you will have a guideline to follow. Some of you might not need this, but most will enjoy the information and guidance. You can purchase the complete programs online for as little as $15 a month, and you will have a fitness trainer assigned to you who will check up on you and your progress.

"When progress is measured it improves, when it is measured and reported back the rate of improvement accelerates."

—Thomas S. Monson

It is important for you to have someone to whom you report your progress, whether it is one of our trainers, or a friend that is also doing the Challenge. Go to wave4life.com if you want to purchase the entire program and get a coach to help you.

The programs are designed with the following individuals in mind:

Level 1 = Beginner

Designed for those with no previous exercise program or activity in their lives and consider themselves to be "beginner" in their fitness goals and objectives.

Level 2 = Intermediate

Designed for those who have had intermittent exercise or activity over the years and consider themselves to be "intermediate" in their fitness goals and objectives.

Level 3 = Advanced

Designed for those who have had consistent exercise or activity over the years and consider themselves "advanced" in their fitness goals and objectives.

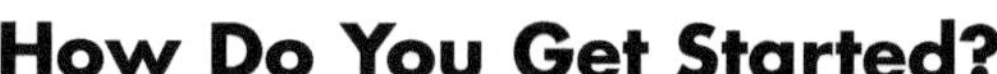

How Do You Get Started?

The first place to start is with the Fitness Evaluation. It is so important to "measure your progress" and get a true starting point. Some say, "I'll complete the Fitness Evaluation when I lose some weight, or get stronger, or start to get in shape", but the problem with this is if you don't measure your progress, you will likely quit before you ever get started. "When progress is measured it improves." This is one of the main things that will motivate you to stick with it, seeing your progress.

So, complete the Fitness Evaluation information today if possible. If you cannot do everything today that is OK, do what you can and fill out the rest ASAP.

If you want to do more than what we have in the Appendix as far as fitness tests go, just do a Google search online for home fitness tests and you will be able to test yourself to your heart's content.

Physical Examination: *It is suggested that you visit your physician for a complete physical examination before starting any exercise program. It is also good to get your blood work done so you can determine what your "inward health" is also.*

On To the Programs

The next step is to get right into the programs and what you will be doing each day. We have designed 3 different activities for you to do each day, an aerobic workout, an anaerobic workout, and a sport or activity workout. You can pick and choose which of the three you want to do each day. You can do more than one daily, but we are not asking for it, we are only asking for 15 – 30 minutes a day in this 6-Week Challenge.

Our goal with the Challenge is to provide an enjoyable routine for you and get you in the habit of exercise, so you will continue to do it after you have completed the Challenge. Be careful of getting all

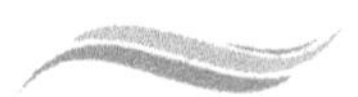

excited about exercise and being fit but having too tough of a routine, you need something that you can sustain for the rest of your life, ease into your exercise routine and make it an enjoyable way of life.

- **Aerobic** – most people know what aerobic exercise is, basically you are getting your heart rate up for a period of time; anything longer than about 45 seconds is considered to be aerobic exercise. Walking, biking, swimming, running, aerobics classes, etc. are all considered to be aerobic exercise.
- **Anaerobic** – some people know what anaerobic exercise is, it is anything less than 45 seconds, things like strength training; lifting weights, doing push-ups, sit-ups, etc.
- **Sport or Activity** – any sport or activity would qualify in which you are getting some form of exercise. Watching sport does not qualify. Yard work, playing basketball, softball, golf, tennis, cleaning the house, walking up and down stairs at work...all of these qualify.
- **When you have finished the Challenge** - Once you have completed our 6–Week Challenge we would like you to let us know you finished it! We want to put your name on the list of people who have completed the Challenge, we would also like any comments *you might have about how you feel, the progress you have made, etc., and if there is any way we can make the Challenge better. Email us at* QETommy@icloud.com

WARNING: Neither tom wright, wave international, wave fitness, nor any of its affiliate companies, officers, personal trainers, independent contractors, or employees are responsible for any advice given here. it is the sole responsibility of each and every person to make sure their workouts are safe and will help them become healthier.

LEVEL 1 - BEGINNER

(rest if needed/tired, in between exercises)

1. Aerobic 6-Days-A-Week – 6-Week Challenge

A. Walking

Day #1 - Walk 5 min.

Day #2 – Walk 5-10 min.

Day #3 – Walk 10-15 min.

Day #4 - Walk 5 min.

Day #5 – Walk 5-10 min.

Day #6 - Walk 10-15 min.

B. Biking

Day #1 - Bike 5 min.

Day #2 – Bike 5-10 min.

Day #3 – Bike 10-15 min.

Day #4 - Bike 5 min.

Day #5 – Bike 5-10 min.

Day #6 – Bike 10-15 min.

C. Other – Do what you like to do. If you like to go to the gym and do your aerobic exercise on the elliptical machine do that. If you like to swim, do that. Remember, anything where you get your heart rate up for more than 45 seconds is considered aerobic exercise.

2. Anaerobic 6-Days-A-Week – 6-Week Challenge

(see online for correct form)

Day #1 – Deadlifts - 10-15 min. total

Set #1 – 20 reps

Set #2 – 20 reps

Set #3 – 20 reps

Day #2 – Push-ups - 10-15 min. total
(on knees or regular)

Set #1 – 10 reps

Set #2 – 10 reps

Set #3 – 10 reps

Day #3 – Squats - 10-15 min. total
(do them with just your body weight)

Set #1 – 20 reps

Set #2 – 20 reps

Set #3 – 20 reps

Day #4 – Shoulder Press *(with 2 cans of soup)* **- 10-15 min. total**

Set #1 – 20 reps

Set #2 – 20 reps

Set #3 – 20 reps

Day #5 – Stomach Crunch 10-15 min. total

Set #1 – 20 reps

Set #2 – 20 reps

Set #3 – 20 reps

Day #6 – Arms Curls with 2 cans of soup – 10-15 min. total

Set #1 – 20 reps

Set #2 – 20 reps

Set #3 – 20 reps

NOTE: Keep your workout challenging enough to be interesting. If cans of soup are too light, find something around the house that weights a little more and use that. Or buy hand weights.

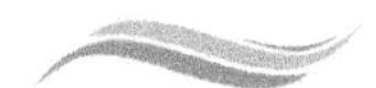

3. Sport or Activity 6-Days-A-Week – 6-Week Challenge

A. Whatever it is you like to do. This might include basketball, softball, working in your yard, golf, tennis, building something, anything physical.

Day #1 – 5-10 min.

Day #2 – 10-15 min.

Day #3 – 15-20 min.

Day #4 – 5-10 min.

Day #5 – 10-15 min.

Day #6 – 15-20 min.

SPECIAL NOTE: Make sure you STRETCH DAILY. The best time to do stretching is *after* your workout because your muscles are loose and warm, so you will be able to push them a lot further then you can before your workout.

LEVEL 2 – INTERMEDIATE

(rest if needed or in between exercises)

1. Aerobic 6-Days-A-Week – 6-Week Challenge

A. Walking

Day #1 - Walk 15 min.

Day #2 – Walk up & down stairs for 5-10 min.

Day #3 – Walk up and down slight hills 15 min

Day #4 - Walk large hill for 10-15 min.

Day #5 – Walk 20 min.

Day #6 - Walk up & down stairs for 10-15 min.

B. Biking

Day #1 – Bike 15 min.

Day #2 – Bike up large hill 5 - 10 min.

Day #3 – Bike up and down slight hills 15 min

Day #4 – Bike up large hill for 10-15 min.

Day #5 – Bike 20 min.

Day #6 – Bike up and down slight hills 10-15 min.

C. Other – Do what you like to do! If you like to go to the gym and do your aerobic exercise on the elliptical machine do that. If you like to swim, do that. Remember, anything where you get your heart rate up for more than 45 seconds is considered aerobic exercise.

2. Anaerobic 6-Days-A-Week – 6-Week Challenge *(see online for correct form)*

Day #1 – Dead lifts *(20-30 min. total)*
Set #1 – 20 reps of light weight to warm-up

Set #2 – 15 reps of light weight

Set #3 – 12 reps of medium weight

Day #2 – Bench Press & Rows - 3 sets of each exercise *(20-30 min. total)*
Set #1 – 20 reps of light weight to warm-up

Set #2 – 15 reps of light weight

Set #3 – 12 reps of medium weight

Day #3 – Squats *(20-30 min. total)*
Set #1 – 20 reps of light weight to warm-up

Set #2 – 15 reps of light weight

Set #3 – 12 reps of medium weight

Day #4 – Shoulder Press & Pull Downs - 3 sets of each exercise *(20-30 min. total)*
Set #1 – 20 reps of lightweight to warm-up

Set #2 – 15 reps of light weight

Set #3 – 12 reps of medium weight

Day #5 – Stomach - 3 sets of 3 different exercises *(10-15 min. total)*

Set #1 – 33 reps of 1st exercise

Set #2 – 33 reps of 2nd exercise

Set #3 – 33 reps of 3rd exercise

Day #6 – Arms - 3 sets each of Biceps & Triceps *(20-30 min. total)*

Set #1 – 20 reps of lightweight to warm up

Set #2 – 15 reps of light weight

Set #3 – 12 reps of medium weight

3. Sport or Activity 6-Days-A-Week – 6-Week Challenge

A. Whatever it is you like to do. This might include basketball,softball, working in your yard, golf, tennis, building something, anything physical.

Day #1 – 10-15 min.

Day #2 – 15-20 min.

Day #3 – 20-30 min.

Day #4 - 10-15 min.

Day #5 – 20 min.

Day #6 - 10-30 min.

SPECIAL NOTE: Make sure you STRETCH DAILY! The best time to do stretching is AFTER your workout because your muscles are loose and warm, so you will be able to push them a lot further then you can before your workout.

LEVEL 3 - ADVANCED

(rest if needed or in between exercises)

1. Aerobic 6-Days-A-Week – 6 Week Challenge

A. Walking

Day #1 - Walk 15 - 30 min.

Day #2 – Walk up & down stairs for 15 - 30 min.

Day #3 – Walk up and down slight hills 30 min.

Day #4 - Walk large hill for 20-30 minutes

Day #5 – Walk 30 min.

Day #6 - Walk up & down stairs for 30 min.

B. Biking

Day #1 - Bike 15 - 30 min.

Day #2 – Bike up large hill 15 - 30 min.

Day #3 – Bike up and down slight hills 30 min

Day #4 - Bike up large hill for 20-30 minutes

Day #5 – Bike 30 min

Day #6 – Bike up and down slight hills 30 min.

C. Other – Do what you like to do. If you like to go to the gym and do your aerobic exercise on the elliptical machine do that. If you like to swim, do that. Remember, anything where you get your heart rate up for more than 45 seconds is considered aerobic exercise.

2. Anaerobic 6-Days-A-Week – 6-Week Challenge *(see online for correct form)*

Day #1 – Dead lifts *(20-30 min. total)*

Set #1 – 12 reps of lightweight to warm-up

Set #2 – 10 reps of medium weight

Set #3 – 10 reps of medium weight

Day #2 – Bench Press & Rows - 3 sets of each exercise *(20-30 min. total)*

Set #1 – 12 reps of lightweight to warm-up

Set #2 – 10 reps of medium weight

Set #3 – 10 reps of medium weight

Day #3 – Squats (20-30 min. total)

Set #1 – 12 reps of lightweight to warm-up

Set #2 – 10 reps of medium weight

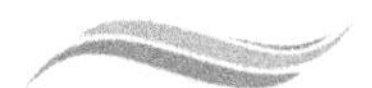

Set #3 – 10 reps of medium weight

Day #4 – Shoulder Press & Pull Downs - 3 sets of each exercise *(20-30 min. total)*

Set #1 – 12 reps of lightweight to warm-up

Set #2 – 10 reps of medium weight

Set #3 – 10 reps of medium weight

Day #5 – Stomach - 3 sets of 3 different exercises *(10-15 min. total)*

Set #1 – 33 reps of 1st exercise

Set #2 – 33 reps of 2nd exercise

Set #3 – 33 reps of 3rd exercise

Day #6 – Arms - 3 sets each of Biceps & Triceps *(20-30 min. total)*

Set #1 – 12 reps of lightweight to warm up

Set #2 – 10 reps of medium weight

Set #3 – 10 reps of medium weight

3. Sport or Activity 6-Days-A-Week – 6-Week Challenge

A. Whatever it is you like to do. This might include basketball, softball, working in your yard, golf, tennis, building something, anything physical.

Day #1 – 15-30 min.

Day #2 – 20-30 min.

Day #3 – 30 min.

Day #4 - 10-20 min.

Day #5 – 30 min.

Day #6 - 15-30 min.

SPECIAL NOTE: Make sure you STRETCH DAILY! The best time to do stretching is AFTER your workout because your muscles are loose and warm, so you will be able to push them a lot further then you can before your workout.

QUESTION EVERYTHING?
GRANDPA, HOW COME WE HAVE PENNIES IF THEY WON'T BUY ANYTHING?
QETommy.com

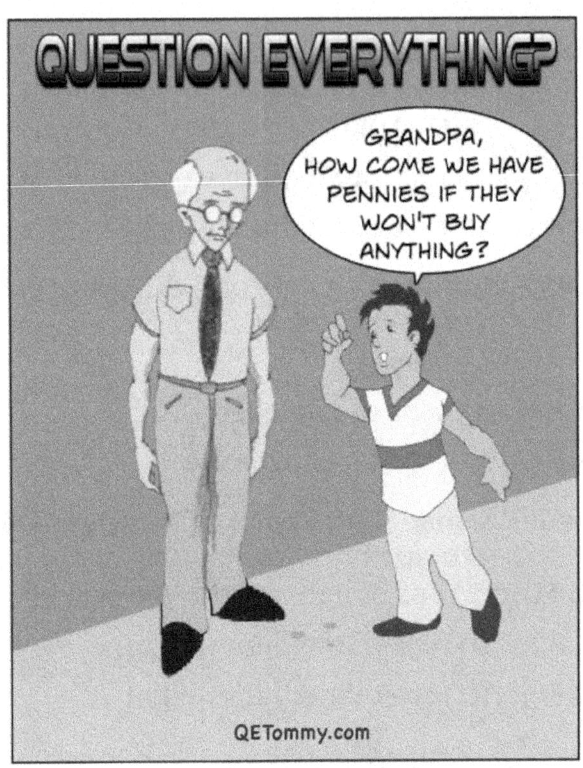

Check-off Sheets

Here is your check off sheets for each week; *put a big check mark when completed.* One (Aerobic, Anaerobic, or Sport or Activity) per day. Also note how you feel. Don't worry if you do not do all 6 workouts in 1 week, check off 1 day at a time until you are finished.

Week #1

Day	Aerobic	Anaerobic	Sport or Activity	Notes
1				
2				
3				
4				
5				
6				

Week #2

Day	Aerobic	Anaerobic	Sport or Activity	Notes
13				
14				
15				
16				
17				
18				

Week #3

Day	Aerobic	Anaerobic	Sport or Activity	Notes
19				
20				
21				
22				
23				
24				

Week #4

Day	Aerobic	Anaerobic	Sport or Activity	Notes
25				
26				
27				
28				
29				
30				

Week #5

Day	Aerobic	Anaerobic	Sport or Activity	Notes
25				
26				
27				
28				
29				
30				

Week #6

Day	Aerobic	Anaerobic	Sport or Activity	Notes
31				
32				
33				
34				
35				
36				

QUESTION EVERYTHING?
HEY MOM, WERE DOES THE SOCK GO WHEN YOU LOSE IT?
QETommy.com

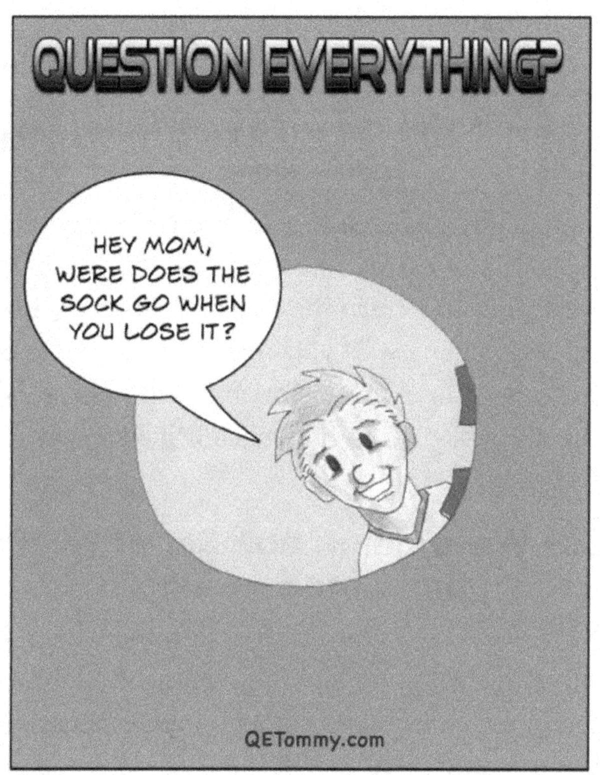

WAVE FOR NUTRITION ANALYSIS

*"When performance is measured it improves,
when performance is measured and reported back
the rate of improvement accelerates."*

—Thomas Monson

Over the past several years we have developed an easy 10-Step Nutritional Analysis that will help you determine your personal nutritional strengths and weaknesses. It will give you suggestions on healthful alternatives to poor food choices, and get you in the habit of healthy nutrition. We use the government's Food Pyramid as the model, with a few changes; the WAVE Food Pyramid.

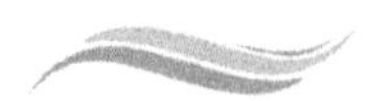

If you need help and support filling this out and sticking to your new nutritional program, visit us on the web at wave4life.com and hire a registered dietitian or coach to help you through the process.

STEP #1 – Write down everything you eat for 1 week.

Do not make any changes to your nutrition program your first week. Your patterns of eating have been established over years and years. We are trying to determine these habits so we can help you make the necessary changes. If you changing the way you have eaten for years, we do not have a true starting point, and this is a critical factor to your success. So, be honest, tell it like it is, and you can change next week.

STEP #2 – Write down number of servings for the 6 food groups.

Use the WAVE Food Pyramid to determine which of the 6 food groups your food fits into. For serving size see the following list. You do not need to be exact. We are looking for general patterns here, not exact numbers of grams, etc.

Serving Size Examples:

- 1 Piece of Bread = 1 Serving of Grains/etc.
- 1 full Corn on the Cob = 2 Servings of Vegetables
- 1 Whole Apple = 2 Servings of Fruit
- 1 small Handful of Nuts = 1 Serving of Nuts
- 1 Cup of Milk = 1 Serving of Milk/Dairy
- 1 Small Candy Bar = 1 Serving of Sweets
- 1 small Bowl of Cereal = 1 Serving of Grains/etc.
- Broccoli and Carrots (1 Cup) = 2 Servings of Vegetables
- ½ Grapefruit = 1 Serving of Fruits
- ½ Pound of Steak = 2 Servings of Meat

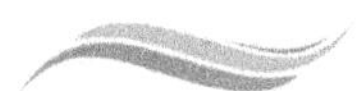

- 1 Large Yogurt = 2 Servings of Milk/Dairy
- 1 Can of Pop (Regular) = 2 Servings of Sweets

NOTE: Before you start copy 2 more additional weeks of the following pages, so you can record a total of 3 weeks of your nutrition.

WEEK #1

SUNDAY

BREAKFAST –

Grains/Vegetables/Fruit/ Beans/Meat/Milk/Dairy Fats/Sweets

SNACK –

Grains/Vegetables/Fruit/ Beans/Meat/Milk/Dairy Fats/Sweets

LUNCH –

Grains/Vegetables/Fruit/ Beans/Meat/Milk/Dairy Fats/Sweets

SNACK –

Grains/Vegetables/Fruit/ Beans/Meat/Milk/Dairy Fats/Sweets

DINNER –

Grains/Vegetables/Fruit/ Beans/Meat/Milk/Dairy Fats/Sweets

SNACK –

Grains/Vegetables/Fruit/ Beans/Meat/Milk/Dairy Fats/Sweetsg

DAILY TOTALS

Grains/Vegetables/Fruit/ Beans/Meat/Milk/Dairy Fats/Sweets

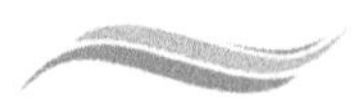

MONDAY

BREAKFAST –

Grains/Vegetables/Fruit/ Beans/Meat/Milk/Dairy Fats/Sweets

SNACK –

Grains/Vegetables/Fruit/ Beans/Meat/Milk/Dairy Fats/Sweets

LUNCH –

Grains/Vegetables/Fruit/ Beans/Meat/Milk/Dairy Fats/Sweets

SNACK –

Grains/Vegetables/Fruit/ Beans/Meat/Milk/Dairy Fats/Sweets

DINNER –

Grains/Vegetables/Fruit/ Beans/Meat/Milk/Dairy Fats/Sweets

SNACK –

Grains/Vegetables/Fruit/ Beans/Meat/Milk/Dairy Fats/Sweets

DAILY TOTALS

Grains/Vegetables/Fruit/ Beans/Meat/Milk/Dairy Fats/Sweets

TUESDAY

BREAKFAST –

Grains/Vegetables/Fruit/ Beans/Meat/Milk/Dairy Fats/Sweets

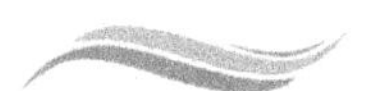

SNACK –

Grains/Vegetables/Fruit/ Beans/Meat/Milk/Dairy Fats/Sweets

LUNCH –

Grains/Vegetables/Fruit/ Beans/Meat/Milk/Dairy Fats/Sweets

SNACK –

Grains/Vegetables/Fruit/ Beans/Meat/Milk/Dairy Fats/Sweets

DINNER –

Grains/Vegetables/Fruit/ Beans/Meat/Milk/Dairy Fats/Sweets

SNACK –

Grains/Vegetables/Fruit/ Beans/Meat/Milk/Dairy Fats/Sweets

DAILY TOTALS

Grains/Vegetables/Fruit/ Beans/Meat/Milk/Dairy Fats/Sweets

WEDNESDAY

BREAKFAST –

Grains/Vegetables/Fruit/ Beans/Meat/Milk/Dairy Fats/Sweets

SNACK –

Grains/Vegetables/Fruit/ Beans/Meat/Milk/Dairy Fats/Sweets

LUNCH –

Grains/Vegetables/Fruit/ Beans/Meat/Milk/Dairy Fats/Sweets

SNACK –

Grains/Vegetables/Fruit/ Beans/Meat/Milk/Dairy Fats/Sweets

DINNER –

Grains/Vegetables/Fruit/ Beans/Meat/Milk/Dairy Fats/Sweets

SNACK –

Grains/Vegetables/Fruit/ Beans/Meat/Milk/Dairy Fats/Sweets

DAILY TOTALS

Grains/Vegetables/Fruit/ Beans/Meat/Milk/Dairy Fats/Sweets

THURSDAY

BREAKFAST –

Grains/Vegetables/Fruit/ Beans/Meat/Milk/Dairy Fats/Sweets

SNACK –

Grains/Vegetables/Fruit/ Beans/Meat/Milk/Dairy Fats/Sweets

LUNCH –

Grains/Vegetables/Fruit/ Beans/Meat/Milk/Dairy Fats/Sweets

SNACK –

Grains/Vegetables/Fruit/ Beans/Meat/Milk/Dairy Fats/Sweets

DINNER –

Grains/Vegetables/Fruit/ Beans/Meat/Milk/Dairy Fats/Sweets

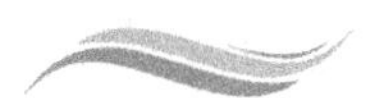

SNACK –

Grains/Vegetables/Fruit/ Beans/Meat/Milk/Dairy Fats/Sweets

DAILY TOTALS:

Grains/Vegetables/Fruit/ Beans/Meat/Milk/Dairy Fats/Sweets

FRIDAY

BREAKFAST –

Grains/Vegetables/Fruit/ Beans/Meat/Milk/Dairy Fats/Sweets

SNACK –

Grains/Vegetables/Fruit/ Beans/Meat/Milk/Dairy Fats/Sweets

LUNCH –

Grains/Vegetables/Fruit/ Beans/Meat/Milk/Dairy Fats/Sweets

SNACK –

Grains/Vegetables/Fruit/ Beans/Meat/Milk/Dairy Fats/Sweets

DINNER –

Grains/Vegetables/Fruit/ Beans/Meat/Milk/Dairy Fats/Sweets

SNACK –

Grains/Vegetables/Fruit/ Beans/Meat/Milk/Dairy Fats/Sweets

DAILY TOTALS:

Grains/Vegetables/Fruit/ Beans/Meat/Milk/Dairy Fats/Sweets

SATURDAY

BREAKFAST –

Grains/Vegetables/Fruit/ Beans/Meat/Milk/Dairy Fats/Sweets

SNACK –

Grains/Vegetables/Fruit/ Beans/Meat/Milk/Dairy Fats/Sweets

LUNCH –

Grains/Vegetables/Fruit/ Beans/Meat/Milk/Dairy Fats/Sweets

SNACK –

Grains/Vegetables/Fruit/ Beans/Meat/Milk/Dairy Fats/Sweets

DINNER –

Grains/Vegetables/Fruit/ Beans/Meat/Milk/Dairy Fats/Sweets

SNACK –

Grains/Vegetables/Fruit/ Beans/Meat/Milk/Dairy Fats/Sweets

DAILY TOTALS:

Grains/Vegetables/Fruit/ Beans/Meat/Milk/Dairy Fats/Sweets

Animal Fats and Sweets Sparingly

1-2 *Organic* Soy Milk, Rice Milk
0-1 *Organic* Non-Fat Milk,
Yogurt, or Cheese

2-3 *Organic* Beans, Nuts & Seeds
0-1 *Organic* Meat, Poultry, Fish, Egg

2-5 Organic Fruit (Instead of sugar)

3-6 Organic Vegetables (Preferably raw or steamed)

4-6 Servings of Organic Whole Wheat Bread,
Pasta & Rice

WAVE FOOD PYRAMID

STEP #4 – Compare your totals to the WAVE Food Pyramid.

Obviously, the totals will vary depending on the size of the individual and his or her activity levels. The recommended servings are for AVERAGE individuals. If you are a large man with a high activity level, you should eat more servings than average. If you are a small woman with little or no activity level, you should eat fewer servings than average. The WAVE Food Pyramid determines general eating habits, deficiencies, and over-indulgences. If you are way out of line with The WAVE Food Pyramid, please consider revising your nutrition so you can live a healthier, happier life.

STEP #5 – Highlight good food choices.

Take a yellow highlighter and highlight all your really good food choices...pat yourself on the back! You did great here, celebrate your successes. Treat yourself to a nice dinner, go to a movie, sit in a Jacuzzi, get a massage, reward yourself. Feel proud of the good choices you make.

STEP #6 – Mark the bad choices.

Use a red pen or pencil. Do not beat yourself up. Just remember where you went wrong so you can do better next time. We are not looking for perfection, only improvement.

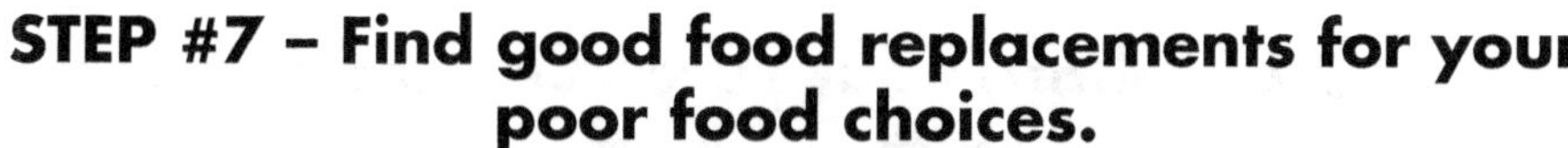

STEP #7 – Find good food replacements for your poor food choices.

The Good	The Bad	The Ugly
Water	Regular Soda	Diet Soda
Fruit	Candy	Fat + Candy
Raw/Steamed	Boiled	Fried
Whole Wheat Bread	White Bread	Donuts
Soy/Rice Milk	Low-Fat Milk	Regular Milk
Fresh Squeezed Juice	Fruit Drinks <100%	Alcohol
Nuts	Nuts + Sugar	Tobacco
Lean Organic Meat	Lean Regular Meat	High Fat Meats
Olive Oil Dressing	Low Cal Dressings	Regular Dressings
Cheese	Low Fat Cheese	Fat Free Cheese
Baked Chips	Low Fat Chips	Regular Chips
Real Butter	Low Fat Spread	Margarine

STEP # 8 – Share your successes and failures with a friend.

"When performance is measured it improves.
When performance is measured and reported back,
the rate of improvement accelerates."

—Thomas Monson

You need someone to report to. Your best friend, someone you are close to, someone who shares your interest in this program, someone who is interested in nutrition...someone who cares about you.

Friend____________________ Phone/ E-mail __________________________

List 2 other friends who would help you:

Friend____________________ Phone/ E-mail __________________________

Friend____________________ Phone/ E-mail __________________________

STEPS #9 & 10 – Chart your progress for 2 more weeks (3 weeks total)

They say it takes 21 days to establish a habit. So, we suggest you track your nutrition at least three weeks. You can do this 3 weeks in a row, or split it up. Maybe once a month for three months, etc. Many people get excited about it all and want to track their nutrition in consecutive weeks. Whichever works best for you.

Congratulations, you have finished! You are doing great; keep the good habits you have established going. If you need help from us logon to wave4life.com and sign up for some coaching.

We appreciate your efforts so very much. Please stay in contact with us at QETommy@icloud.com and let us know how you are doing.

God bless you!

Team WAVE

About the Author

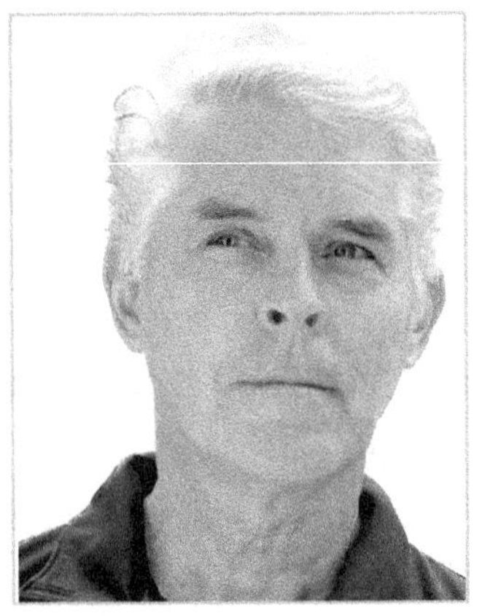

Tom Wright is a professional athlete and health educator. He's a former NY Yankee outfielder, and hosts and produces a TV show about healthy living that has run into over 50 million homes on mainstream television. Thirty plus of the regional TV show episodes are posted on our website, Wave4Life.com

Currently he is working on getting on the Champions (Senior) PGA Tour, and hopes to qualify for the European Senior Tour next year.

Tom has a college degree from Brigham Young University in Physical Education, and started a Masters Program, also in Physical Education, before his offer to play with the Yankees. He has also played in the Mexican Major Leagues, and is now a knuckleball pitcher. Tom is still hoping to pitch in Major League Baseball, and become the only player to ever compete on into his 60's. His fastball is still in the 80's.

Tom has been a competitive power lifter, with a dead lift of over 600 pounds, and a squat of 500 pounds in competition. He's captured on video easily dead lifting 405 pounds four times at age 57.

Tom is also the author of the *Question Everything Comics*, along with illustrator, David Lau. Their first book, *Tommy Goes to the Beach*, is now available and can be purchased online at QETommy. com.

Tom has many other interests and hobbies including art, movies, writing, reading, and classic cars. He's written over 20,000 pages just in his journals.

Tom loves people and is passionate about helping as many people as possible to live healthy and happy lives. .

I have been very blessed in my life to have wonderful parents, great teachers and friends, and opportunities to go to school, play professional sports, and learn many things from people much wiser than myself. The principles taught here are not mine, I believe they come from God, I know things can be better said, and I'm sure I've left some really important things out of this discussion that should be included. Please let me know if you see any major flaws, or feel something should be included in subsequent editions. Write to me at QETommy@icloud.com.

Thank you so much for reading and I hope something I've said might help you in your life.

Sincerely,

Tom Wright

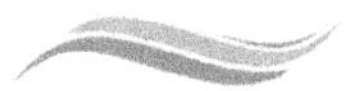

Endnotes

1

REFERENCES

These references are taken from sources that are meant to be studied, mostly from classic books about healthy living. You can visit www.Books.Google.com and read many of these references directly, and oftentimes the entire book is there online for free.

Fitness Section:

1 *FOX News*, November, 2009

2 Packer, B., *Mine Errand from the Lord* 310-311, 2008

3 Golding, L., *Y's Way to Fitness*, 3rd Edition. Appendix, 1989

4 Cooper, K., *Aerobics*, 1968

5 Jakicic, J., Winters, C.,Lang, W., Wing, R., *Effects of Intermittent Exercise and Use of Home Exercise Equipment on Adherence, Weight Loss, and Fitness in Overweight Women, JAMA*, 282:1554-1560, 1999

6 The Doctors Told Me that Stress Caused My... Kansas State University website: http://www.k-state.edu/counseling/topics/stress/drstress.html 1997

7 Young, R., Young, S., *The pH Miracle: Balance Your Diet, Reclaim Your Health, Introduction*, 2002

8 Lockhart, B., *Mind/Body Fitness*, 1992

9 Sinha, A., *Heart Monitor Training*, MarathonGuide.com website: http://www.marathonguide.com/training/articles/HeartMonitorTraining.cfm, 2010

10 Abadjiev, I., *Bulgarian Training Methodology*, http://www.owresource.com/training/bulgarian.php, 2010

11 Kreider, R.B., *Overtraining in Sport*, 1998

12 Chopra, D., *Unconditional Life: Discovering the Power to Fulfill Your Dreams*, 1992

13 Whitmore, J., Costell, D., Kenney, L., *Physiology of Sport and Exercise*, 247, 2008

14 Whitmore, J., Costell, D., Kenney, L., *Physiology of Sport and Exercise*, 189, 2008

15 Schwartzenegger, A., Dobins, B., *The New Encyclopedia of Modern BodyBuilding*, 93, 1998

16 Schwartzenegger, A., Dobins, B., *Arnold's BodyBuilding For Men*, 93, 1984

17 National Association of Basketball Coaches of the United States, American Football Coaches Association, American Football Coaches Association. Meeting, *Athletic Journal*, Volume 55, 62, 1974

18 Vella, M., *Anatomy for Strength and Fitness Training*, 2006

19 Beck, K., *Run Strong*, 2005

20 Katz, A., *The Physiology of the Heart*, 49, 2001

21 Garrett, W., Kirkendall, W., *Exercise and Sport Science*, 698, 2000

22 Cooper, K., *Aerobics*, 1968

23 Taylor, K., *The Book: 21 Day Habit*, 1999

24 Brody, J., *Jane Brody's Good Food Book: Living the high carbohydrate way*, 221, 1985

25 Blake, D., Winyard, P. *Immunopharmacology of Free Radical Species*, 87, 1995

26 Bailey, C., *Smart Exercise: Burning Fat, Getting Fit*, 108, 1995

27 Tsatsouline, P., *Power To The People: Russian Strength Training Secrets for Every American*, 144, 2000

28 Benson, H., Stuart, E. *The Wellness Book*, 110, 1993

29 Williams, T., *Ted Williams: The Pursuit of Perfection*, 227, 2002

30 McGowan, M., Chopra, J., *50 Ways To Lower Cholesterol*, 83, 2002

31 Burke, E., *Precision Heart Rate Training*, 9, 1998

32 Navratilova, M., Douillard, J., *Body Mind and Sport*, 171, 2001

33 Connors, E., Grymkowski, K., *Golds Gym Mass Building Training and Nutrition System*, 203,1992

34 Smolenski, M., Lamberg, L., *Body Clock Guide to Better Health*, 119, 2001

35 Fleck, S., Kraemer, W., *Designing Resistance Training Programs*, 159, 2004

36 Zimbardo, P., *The Cognitive Control of Motivation: The Consequences of Choice and Dissonance*, 269, 1969

37 Shepard, G., *Bigger, Faster, Stronger*, 61, 2004

38 Incledon, L., *Strength Training for Women*, 162, 2005

39 Bird, S., Black, N., Newton, P., Campling, J., *Sports Injuries: Causes, Diagnosis, Treatment, and Prevention*, 123, 1997

40 Foran, B., *High-Performance Sports Conditioning*, 27, 2001

41 Price, R., *The Ultimate Guide to Weight Training for Golf*, 83, 2003

42 Berger, K., *The Developing Person Through the Life Span*, 418, 2004

43 Lawrence, R., Zuckler, M., *Preventing Arthritis: A Holistic Approach to Life Without Pain*, 75, 2002

44 Drucker, S., Cathcart, R., *American Heroes in a Media Age*, 236, 1994

45 Famighetti, R., *World Almanac and Book Facts*, 43, 1996

46 2009 Open Championship, Turnberry, Scottland

47 Sleamaker, R., Browning, R., *Serious Training for Endurance Athletes*, 81,1996

48 Wolff, R., *BodyBuilding 101: Everything You Need to Know to Get The Body You Want*, 9, 1999

49 Kempter, S., *How Muscles Learn: Teaching The Violin With the Body in Mind*, 2003

50 Bompa, T., Carrera, M., *Periodization Training for Sports*, 46, 2005

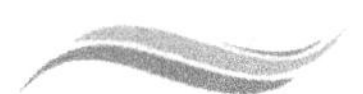

51 Draovich, P., Simpson, R. *Complete Conditioning for Golf*, 23, 2007

52 Blahnik, J., *Full-Body Flexibility*, 8, 2004

53 Tsatsouline, P., *Power To The People: Russian Strength Training Secrets for Every American*, 22, 2000

54 Donatelli, R., *Sports-Specific Rehabilitation*, 321, 2007

55 Stephano, M., *The Firefighters Workout Book*, 20, 2001

56 Connally, C., *The Mountaineering Handbook*, 287, 2004

57 Salvo, S., *Massage Therapy, Principles and Practice*, 559, 1999

58 Smith, B., *The Power Within Us, Ensign Magazine*, 58, Feb. 1983

59 Kelly, T., *Healing The Broken Mind: Transforming America's Failed Mental Health Care System*, 2009

60 Scott, R., *Peace of Conscious and Peace of Mind, Liahona Magazine*, 15-18, Nov. 2004

NUTRITION SECTION:

61 WAVE Mission - Teach as many people as possible true and correct principles of healthy living in a fun and interesting way, and help them to live life optimally, Body, Mind and Spirit.

62 John 8:32

63 Weisse, A, *The Staff and The Serpent: Pertinent and Impertinent Observations of the World of Medicine*, 45, 1998

64 Armstrong, K., *A History of God: From Abraham to the Present, the 4,000 Year Quest for God*, 68, 1993

65 Tomassi, P., *Logic*, 1999

66 Silvester, L., *Weight Training for Strength and Fitness*, 1992

67 Day, L., *Double Blind: What Science Can't See*, www.DrDay.com, 2009

68 Brown, J., Isaacs, J., Brinke, U., *Nutrition Through the Life Cycle*, 2007

69 Sorenson, M., *Mega Health*, 33, 1992

70 Deville, N., *Death By Supermarket: The Fattening, Dumbing Down, and Poisoning of America*, 215, 2007

71 Schwartzenegger, A., Dobins, B., *The New Encyclopedia of Modern BodyBuilding*, 93, 1998

72 Steinn, J. Pruit, B., *Decisions for Healthy Living*, 18, 2003

73 *Business Week Magazine*, Issues 3886-3889, 12, 2004

74 Matcha, D., *Healthcare Systems of the Developed World: How the United States System Remains and Outlier*, 17, 2003

75 CIA, *The CIA World Factbook*, 109, 2008

76 U.S. Senate, Congress, Committee on Finance, *What's Driving Healthcare Costs and the Uninsured: Hearings*, 116, 2004

77 Roehrig, C., Miller, G., Hughes-Cromwick, P., Lake, C., *Quantifying National*

Spending on Wellness and Prevention, Altarum Institute, 2008, http://www.ncbi.nlm.nih.gov/pubmed/19548511

78 Barefoot, R., Reich, C., *The Calcium Factor: The Scientific Secret of Health and Youth*, 2002

79 Allen, J., *Heart Disease to Cost U.S. $503 Billion in 2010, Reuters*, U.S., December, 2009 http://www.reuters.com/article/idUSTRE5BG52I20091217

80 Belle, G., Fisher, L., *Biostatistics: A Methodology for the Health Sciences*, 726, 2004

81 Ornish, Dean, *Dr. Dean Ornish's Program for Reversing Heart Disease: The Only System Scientifically Proven to Reverse Heart Disease without Drugs*, 1991

82 Campbell, T.Colin, Campbell, T., *The China Study: The Most Comprehensive Study of Nutrition Ever Conducted*, 15, 2005

83 Nathanson, C., *Disease Prevention as Social Change: The State, Society and Public Health in United States, France, Great Britain, and Canada*, 2007

84 Kita, J., *Fighting Fat Around the World, Readers Digest Magazine*, 2010, http://shine.yahoo.com/channel/health/fighting-fat-around-the-world-567295/

85 Ornish, Dean, *Dr. Dean Ornish's Program for Reversing Heart Disease: The Only System Scientifically Proven to Reverse Heart Disease without Drugs*, 1991

86 Moody, H., *Concepts and Controversies*, 170, 2009

87 Hearing Before the Committee on The Budget, House of Representatives, Second Session, 42, February 14th, 2006

88 Barefoot, R., Reich, C., *The Calcium Factor: The Scientific Secret of Health and Youth*, 2002

89 Roehrig, C., Miller, G., Hughes-Cromwick, P., Lake, C., *Quantifying National Spending on Wellness and Prevention*, Altarum Institute, 2008, http://www.ncbi.nlm.nih.gov/pubmed/19548511

90 Taylor, E., Brantly, E., *Creating Success from the Inside Out: Develop the Focus and Strategy to Undercover the Life You Want*, 57, 2007

91 Birney, R., Burdick, H., Teevan, R., *Fear of Failure*, 1969

92 Webster, E., *The Fear of Success: Stop It From Stopping You*, 1996

93 Ferrera, L., *Body Mass Index: New Research*, 226

94 Clark, M., NASM, Lucett, S., Corn, R., *NASM Essentials of Personal Fitness Training*, 114, 2007

95 Misra, S., Yadav,. P., *International Business: Text and Cases*, 276, 2009

96 http://www.nuskin.com/nuskin/us/en/products/pharmanex1/scanner.html

97 Friedman, T., *Comparison of Test Methods Used to Access Competence in the Health Fields*, 1986

98 Heymsfield, S., *Human Body Composition*, 29, 2005

99 Bauer, J., *The Complete Idiots Guide to Total Nutrition*, 214, 2005

100 www.thecompetitiveedge.com

101 Perry, J., *Hip To Be Fit: How to Improve Your Physical, Mental, and Financial Health in Under 10 Minutes,* 162, 2008

102 Coulter, C., *Blindside*, 132, 2004

103 Challem, J., Werback, M., *The Food-Mood Solution: All-Natural Ways to Banish Anxiety, Depression, Anger, Stress, Overeating, and Alcohol and Drug Problems, and Feel Good Again*, 13, 2007

104 Koenig, H., McConnell, M., *The Healing Power of Faith: How Belief and Prayer Can Help You Triumph Over Disease*, 72, 2001

105 Michaels, J., Darwin, C., Van Aalst, M., *Master Your Metabolism: The 3 Diet Secrets To Naturally Balance Your Hormones For a Hot and Healthy Body*, 148, 2009

106 Gropper, S., Smith, J., Groff, J., *Advanced Nutrition and Human Metabolism*, 226, 2005

107 Wilmore, J., Costell, D., Kenney, K., *Physiology of Sport and Exercise*, 49, 2008

108 Fuhrman, J., *Eat To Live: The Revolutionary Formula For Fast and Sustained Weight Loss*, 92, 2005

109 Kassirer J., Angell M., *Losing Weight - an ill fated New Years resolution, N. Engl J Med* 1998; 338: 52-4

110 Cruise, J., *The 3-Hour Diet: How Low-Carb Diets Make You Fat and Timing Makes You Thin*, 2005

111 Sorenson, M., *Mega Health*, 36, 1992

112 American Dietetic Association, Duyff, R., *American Dietetic Association Complete Food and Nutrition Guide*, 461, 2006

113 American Medical Association, *JAMA: The Journal of the American Medical Association*, Volume 34, 729, 1900

114 Donald, R., *Turn Your Body Into a Fat Burning Machine Without Strenuous Exercise*, 2007

115 Carlson, K., Eisenstat, S., Ziporan, T., *The New Harvard Guide to Women's Health*, 43, 2004

116 Whitaker, L., Davis, W., *The Bulimic College Student: Evaluation, Treatment, and Prevention*, 135, 1989

117 Sorenson, M., *Mega Health*, 376, 1992

118 Dalton, S., *Overweight and Weight Management: The Health Professional's Guide to Understanding and Practice*, 128, 1997

119 Hofmekler, O., Gallagher, M., *Maximum Muscle, Minimum Fat*, 8, 2008

120 Cruise, J., *The 3-Hour Diet: How Low Carb Diets Make You Fat and Timing Makes You Thin*, 2005

121 Willcox, B., Willcox, C., *The Okinawa Program: How the World's Longest-Lived People Achieve Everlasting Health--and How You Can Too*, 50, 201

122 Balch, P., *Prescription for Nutritional Healing*, 6, 2006

123 *Health*, Volume 21, 146, 1989

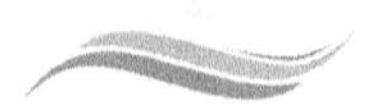

124 Sears, B., *A Week in the Zone*, 2004

125 Graham, D., 80-10-10 *Diet: Balancing Your Health, Your Weight, and Your Life One Luscious Bite at a Time*, 2006

126 Campbell, T.Colin, Campbell, T., *The China Study: The Most Comprehensive Study of Nutrition Ever Conducted*, 85-87, 2005

127 Day, L., *Conquering Confusion About Your Medical Treatment*, 2001

128 Genesis 9:3, Deuteronomy 12:15, 1 Timothy 4:3

129 Campbell, T.Colin, Campbell, T., *The China Study: The Most Comprehensive Study of Nutrition Ever Conducted*, 308-309, 2005

130 Hegsted, D., *Minimum Protein Requirements of Adults, American Journal of Clinical Nutrition*, 21:3520, 1968

131 Fuhrman, J., *Eat To Live: The Revolutionary Formula for Fast and Sustained Weight Loss*, 139, 2005

132 King, I., Schuler, L., *Men's Health, The Book of Muscle: The World's Most Authoritative Guide To Building Your Body*, 44, 2003

133 USDA National Nutrient Database for Standard Reference Legacy (2018)

134 Cox, P., *You Don't Need Meat*, 2003

135 Robbins, J., *Healthy at 100: The Scientifically Proven Secrets of the World's Healthiest and Long-Lived Peoples*, 123, 2006

136 Edlin, G., Golanty, E., *Health and Wellness*, 102, 2007

137 Fuhrman, J., *Disease Proof Your Child: Feeding Kids Right*, 29, 2006

138 Insel, P., Turner, R., Ross, D., *Discovering Nutrition*, 265, 2009

139 Paulien, G., *The Divine Prescription and Science of Health and Healing*, 222, 1995

140 Slifkin, N., *Man and Beast: Our Relationships with Animals in Jewish Law and Thought*, 174, 2006

141 Balch, P., *Prescription for Nutritional Healing*, 3, 2006

142 Strathern, P., *A Brief History of Medicine: From Hippocrates to Gene Therapy*, 2005

143 Barefoot, R., Reich, C., *The Calcium Factor: The Scientific Secret of Health and Youth*, 24, 2002

144 *British Medical Journal: BMJ*, Volume 1, 33, 1956

145 Silvester, L., *Weight Training for Strength and Fitness*, 1992

146 *British Medical Journal* 1991 (Oct 5): 303: 798-799

147 National Library of Medicine: Five-year survival rates of melanoma patients treated by diet therapy after the manner of Gerson: a retrospective review: GL. Hildenbrand et al. *Altern Ther Health Med*, 1995 Sep.

148 Favier, A., *Analysis of Free Radicals in Biological Systems*, 1995

149 Milbury, P., Richer, A., *Understanding the Antioxidant Controversy: Scrutinizing the "Fountain of Youth"*, 34, 2008

150 McDougal, J. The McDougal Program. 315, 1990

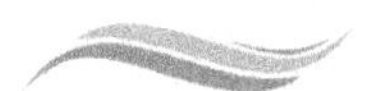

151 Simone, C., *Cancer and Nutrition: A Ten Point Plan for Prevention*, 77, 2005

152 Fuhrman, J., *Eat To Live: The Revolutionary Formula for Fast and Sustained Weight Loss*, 77, 2005

153 Lodish, H., Berk, A., Kaiser, *Molecular Cell Biology*, 1108, 2008

154 Fisher, W., *How To Fight Cancer and Win*, 68, 2003

155 *Virtual Chembook*, Elmerst College, Charles E. Ophardt, c. 2003, pH Scale

156 Miller, D., *Grow Youthful: Ancient Secrets, Modern Research*, 64, 2003

157 Krebs, H., Schmidt, H., *Otto Warburg: Cell Physiologist, Biochemist, and Eccentric*, Clarendon Press, Oxford, 8-9, 1981

158 http://www.3quarksdaily.com/3quarksdaily/2006/07/new_letters_she.html

159 Wikipedia, Otto Heinrich Warburg, http://www.3quarksdaily.com/3quarksdaily/2006/07/new_letters_she.html

160 *The Acid-Alkaline Diet for Optimal Health: Restore Your Health By Creating pH Balance in Your Diet*, 161, 2006

161 Weinstein, R., *The Stress Effect: Discover the Connection Between Stress and Disease and Reclaim Your Health*, 118, 2004

162 Barefoot, R., Reich, C., *The Calcium Factor: The Scientific Secret of Health and Youth*, 67, 2002

163 Wallach, J., *Rare Earths: Forbidden Cures*, 191, 1996

164 Barefoot, R., Reich, C., *The Calcium Factor: The Scientific Secret of Health and Youth*, 67, 2002

165 www.drday.com

166 Mourning, A., Wetzel, D., *Resilience*, 196, 2009

167 Tom's call to American Cancer Society, 2002

168 American Dietetic Association, Duyff, R., *American Dietetic Association Complete Food and Nutrition Guide*, 109, 2006

169 Cadenas, E., Packer, L., *Handbook of Antioxidants*, 594, 2002

170 Gropper, S., Smith, J., Groff, J., *Advanced Nutrition and Human Metabolism*, 122, 2008

171 Servan-Schreiber, D., *Anticancer: A New Way of Life*,

172 Alexander, R., *Victory Over Fat: 6 Steps To Permanent Fat Loss and Super Health*, 78, 2005

173 Alberts, B., *Essential Cell Biology*, 727, 2004

174 Warshawsky, D., Landolph, J., *Molecular Carcinogenesis and the Molecular Biology of Human Cancer*, 134, 2006

175 Brown, S., Trivieri, L., *The Acid-Alkaline Food Guide: A Quick Reference To Foods and Their Effect On pH Levels*, 2006

176 Justice, B., *Think Yourself Healthy: How Thoughts, Moods, and Beliefs Affect Your Health*, 1989

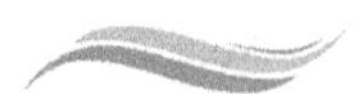

177 Personal Story told to Tom, 2002

178 Young, R., Young, S., *The pH Miracle: Balance Your Diet, Reclaim Your Health*, 2002

179 Harvard Medical School, *Healthy Eating: A Guide To Nutrition*, 13, 2003

180 Block, G., Professor of Epidemiology and Public Health Nutrition at the University of California, Berkeley, March 28, 2007, http://www.sixwise.com/newsletters/07/03/28/the-seven-nutrients-americans-are-most-deficient-in--amp-how-to-get-them.htm

181 Storey, K., *Functional Metabolism: Regulation and Adaptation*, 268, 2004

182 Radak, Z., *Free Radicals in Exercise and Aging*, 1, 2000

183 Weil, A., *Why I Am a Conservative On Healthcare Reform*, August 16, 2009, http://www.huffingtonpost.com/andrew-weil-md/why-i-am-a-conservative-o_b_259869.html

184 U.S. Senate, Congress, Committee on Finance, *What's Driving Healthcare Costs and the Uninsured: Hearings*, 116, 2004

185 Walford, R., *Beyond the 120 Year Diet: How To Double Your Vital Years*, 9, 2000

186 Barefoot, R., Reich, C., *The Calcium Factor: The Scientific Secret of Health and Youth,* xxiv, 2002

187 LaPlace, J., *Health*, 272, 1984

188 Austin, D., *Fit and Fabulous After 40:A 5-Part Program for Turning Back the Clock*, 151, 2002

189 Carlo, G., Schram, M., *Cell Phones: Invisible Hazards in the Wireless Age*, 234, 2002

190 Weil, A., *Spontaneous Healing: How to Discover and Embrace Your body's Natural Ability to Maintain and Heal Itself,* 211, 2000

191 Baker, N., *The Body Toxic: How the Hazardous Chemistry of Everyday Things Threaten Our Health and Well-Being*, 90, 2008

192 Kamhi, E., Zampieron, E., *Arthritis: Reversing Underlying Causes of Arthritis With Clinically Proven Alternative Therapies*, 119, 2006

193 Nies, D., Silver, S., *Molecular Microbiology of Heavy Metals*, 106, 2007

194 Brownstein, D., *Overcoming Arthritis*, 2001

195 Kirby, D., *Evidence of Harm: Mercury in Vaccines and the Autism Epidemic: A Medical Controversy*, 2005

196 Brownstein, D., *Overcoming Arthritis*, 2001

197 Ziff, S., *Silver Dental Fillings: The Toxic Time Bomb: Can The Mercury in Your Dental Fillings Poison You*, 46, 2002

198 Thomas, P., *What's In This Stuff: The Hidden Toxins in Everyday Products and What You Can Do About Them*, 150, 2008

199 Fuhrman, J., *Eat To Live: The Revolutionary Formula for Fast and Sustained Weight Loss*, 13, 2005

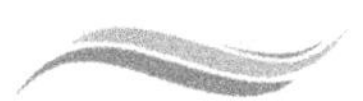

200 Fuhrman, J., *Eat To Live: The Revolutionary Formula for Fast and Sustained Weight Loss*, 195, 2005

201 Fuhrman, J., *Eat To Live: The Revolutionary Formula for Fast and Sustained Weight Loss*, 7, 2005

202 Fuhrman, J., *Eat To Live: The Revolutionary Formula for Fast and Sustained Weight Loss*, 120, 2005

203 Fuhrman, J., *Eat To Live: The Revolutionary Formula for Fast and Sustained Weight Loss*, 304, 2005

204 Packer, B. *Mine Errand from the Lord* 310-311, 2008

205 Smith, E., *The Vegetable Gardner's Bible*, 289, 2004

206 Wallach, J., *Rare Earths: Forbidden Cures*, 171, 1996

207 Uphoff, N., *Biological Approaches to Sustainable Soil Systems*, 19, 2006

208 Nair, P., *An Introduction to Agroforestry*, 66, 1993

209 Wallach, J., *Rare Earths: Forbidden Cures*, 251, 1996

210 Roberts, B., *Land Care Manual*, 102, 1992

211 Weil, A., *8 Weeks to Optimal Health: A Proven Program for Taking Full Advantage of Your Body's Natural Healing Power*, 90, 2007

215 DiSilvestro, R., *Handbook of Minerals as Nutritional Supplements*, 2005

213 http://www.lifezone.com/

214 http://www.purezonenow.com/index_files/Page350.htm

215 Wright, R., Nebel, B., *Environmental Science: The Way The World Works*, 608, 1993

216 http://www.albionminerals.com/

217 http://www.albionminerals.com/knowledge/chelates-not-created-equal?start=1

218 Ashmead, D., *Chelated Mineral Nutrition in Plants, Animals, and Man*, 1982

219 Ashmead, D., Ashmead, H., Graff, D., *Intestinal Absorption of Metal Ions and Chelates*, 13, 1985

220 http://www.albionminerals.com/knowledge/qaa-about-amino-acid-chelates

221 Margolis, S., Johns Hopkins Medical Institutions, T*he Johns Hopkins Complete Home Guide to Symptoms & Remedies*, 36, 2004

222 http://www.albionminerals.com/albion-history

223 Dr. Janeel Henderson, daughter of Founder Dr. Harvey Ashmead, personal conversation, 2006

224 http://www.albionminerals.com/

225 http://www.lifezone.com/

226 Harris, M., *A Culture of Steroid Use of Among High School Athletes*, 117, 2008 http://blog.nj.com/hssportsextra/2009/05/is_states_high_school_steroid.html

227 Barron, J., *Lessons From The Miracle Doctors*, 78, 2002

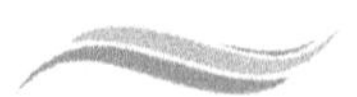

228 Sorenson, M., *Mega Health*, 429-430, 1992

229 Cousins, G., *Spiritual Nutrition: Six Foundations for Spiritual Life and the Awakening of Kundalini,* 258, 2005

230 Wallach, J., *Rare Earths: Forbidden Cures*, 191, 1996

231 Wallach, J., *Rare Earths: Forbidden Cures*, 171, 1996

232 Wallach, J., *Rare Earths: Forbidden Cures*, 191, 1996

233 http://www.totaltucker.com.au/pig.htm

234 Sorrenson, M., *Mega Health*, 1992

235 Spurlock, M, *Super Size Me* Movie, http://en.wikipedia.org/wiki/Super_Size_Me, 2003

236 Hemat, R., *Orthomolecularism: Principles and Practice*, 515, 2004

237 Tom asking Sweet Tomatoes Manager, 2009

238 http://originalfastfoods.com/serendipity/index.php?/archives/4-Jim-and-Colleens-Story.html

239 Find – talk to kids 2-3 min a day

240 Covey, S., *Seven Habits of Highly Effective Families*, 266, 1997

241 Day, L., *Conquering Confusion About Your Medical Treatment*, 2001

242 Fink, H., Burgoon, L., Mikesky, A., *Practical Applications in Sports Nutrition*, 234, 2008

243 Batmanhelidj, F., *Water: For Health, For Healing, For Life: You're Not Sick, You're Thirsty*, 187, 2003

244 American Dietetic Association, Duyff, R., *American Dietetic Association Complete Food and Nutrition Guide*, 572, 2006

245 Starr, C., McMillan, B., *Human Biology*, 2008

246 Hart, C., Grossman, M., *The Insulin-Resistance Diet: How To Turn Off Your Body's Fat-Making Machine*, 60, 2001

247 Boyle, M., Long, S., *Personal Nutrition*, 90, 2006

248 Bagchi, D., Preuss, H., *Obesity: Epidemiology, Pathophysiology, and Prevention*, 249, 2007

249 McCullough, F., *Living Low-Carb: The Complete Guide to Long-Term Low-Carb Dieting*, 3, 2003

250 Rhodes, J., *Fat To Fit Without Dieting*, 202, 1990

251 Wylde, B., *The Antioxidant Prescription: How To Use The Power of Antioxidants to Prevent Disease and Stay Healthy for Life*, 133, 2008

252 Gropper, S., Smith, J., Groff, J., *Advanced Nutrition and Human Metabolism*, 76, 2008

253 *University Health News, Glycemic Index Chart, GI Ratings for Hundreds of Foods*, by Chandra Johnson-Green, June 22, 2020

254 http://www.glycemicedge.com/glycemic-index-chart/

255 Taubes, G., *Good Calories, Bad Calories: Fats, Carbs, and the Controversial Science of Diet and Healt*h, 197, 2008

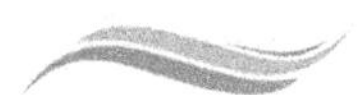

256 Michaels, J., Darwin, C., Van Aalst, M., *Master Your Metabolism: The 3 Diet Secrets To Naturally Balance Your Hormones For a Hot and Healthy Body*, 147, 2009

257 Meyerowitz, S., *The Organic Food Guide: How To Shop Smarter and Healthier*, 39, 2004

258 McGee, H., *On Food and Cooking: The Science and Lore of the Kitchen*, 285, 2004

259 Jellinek, M., Houston, J., *What Should I Feed My Kids: A Pediatricians Guide to Safe and Healthy Food and Growth*, 45, 1996

260 Robbins, J., *Healthy at 100: The Scientifically Proven Secrets of the Worlds Healthiest and Longest-Lived People*, 146, 2007

261 Bauer, J., *The Complete Idiots Guide to Total Nutrition*, 258, 2005

262 Day, L., *Conquering Confusion About Your Medical Treatment*, 2001

263 Paulien, G., *The Divine Prescription and Science of Health and Healing*, 205, 1995, Proverbs 27:27

264 Fuhrman, J., *Eat To Live: The Revolutionary Formula for Fast and Sustained Weight Loss*, 63, 2005

265 Day, L., *Conquering Confusion About Your Medical Treatment*, 2001

266 Sorenson, M., *Mega Health*, 179, 1992

267 Day, L., *Conquering Confusion About Your Medical Treatment*, 2001

268 Saidoff, D., Apfel, S., *The Healthy Body Handbook: A Total Guide to Prevention and Treatment of Sports Injuries*, 300, 2005

269 Pirello, C., *This Crazy Vegan Life: A Prescription for an Endangered Species*, 68, 2008

270 Tribole, E., *The Ultimate Omega-3 Diet: Maximize The Power of Omega 3's to Supercharge Your Health, Battle Inflammation, and Keep Your Mind Sharp*, 182, 2007

271 Sherman, C., *The Best of All Worlds: The Complete Culinary Guide to Feeling Great, Staying Young, and Saving the Earth*, 96, 2003

272 Day, L., *Conquering Confusion About Your Medical Treatment*, 2001

273 May, J., *Miracle of Stevia: Discover the Healing Power of Nature's Herbal Sweetener*, 217, 2003

MIND SECTION:

274 Wilson, S. *Every Woman Dreams Lyrics*

275 Genesis 25:29-34

276 Hill, N., *Think and Grow Rich*, 2005

277 Hill, N. *The Law of Success: In 16 Lessons*, 2000

278 Samadi, A., *The Secret for Teens Revealed*, 199, 2008

279 Losier, M. *Law of Attraction: The Science of Attracting More of What You Want and Less of What You Don't Want*, 2004

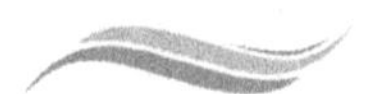

280 *BlackBelt Magazine*, 31, Mar. 1979

281 Little, B., *The Secret and Spirituality*, 125, 2008

282 Wrisberg, C. *Sport Skill Instruction for Coaches*, 59, 2007

283 Rotella, R., Cullen, B. *Golf Is Not A Game of Perfect*, 132, 1995

284 Miller, J., Yocom, G., *I Call The Shots*, 3, 2004

285 Matthew 11:30

286 Kelly, K., *The Secret of The Secret*, 175, 2007

287 Pink, D., *A Whole New Mind: Why Right-Brainers Will Rule The Future*, 203, 2006

288 Warren, D., *Mind Over Time: Feel The Joy of Awakening Infinite Capabilities*, 2006

289 Lawson, S., Holman Old Testament Commentary: Psalms 76-150, 267, 2006

290 Thielicke, H., *The Evangelical Faith, Volume 1*, 86, 1974

291 DeStefano, A., *Ten Prayers God Always Says Yes To*, 171, 2009

292 Koppel, R., *The Intuitive Trader: Developing You Inner Trading Wisdom*, 202, 1996

293 Doctrine and Covenants 58:21

294 Dickens, C., *Great Expectations*, 23, 2003

295 Mosiah 4:27

296 Norhanian, A. *College is for Suckers: The First College Guide You Should Read*, 2009

297 *The National News - Lifestyle, Seven Minutes a Day: the modern-day excuse for a parent*, Clifton Chadwick, Nov. 14, 2011y

298 Tucker, L., *What's On TV Tonight, Ensign*, 18, 1988

299 Lickona, T., *Character Matters: How To Help Our Children Develop Good Judgement, Integrity and Other Essential Virtues*, 189, 2004

300 Kimball, J., *More J Golden Kimball stories*, 2002

301 Bach, D., *Start Late, Finish Rich: A No-Fail Plan for Achieving Financial Freedom at Any Age*, 330, 2007

302 Campbell, C., *The Wealthy Spirit: Daily Affirmations For Financial Stress Reduction*, Introduction, 2002

303 Covey, S., *Seven Habits of Highly Effective Families*, 145, 1997

304 United Nations Development Programme, Human Development Report 2003 (New York: Oxford University Press), 40-41, 2003

305 Steiner, G., Steiner, J., *Business, Government, and Society: A Managerial Perspective: Text and Cases*, 26, 2005

306 Nieto, S., *What Keeps Teachers Going?* 57, 2003

307 Bear, J., Bear, M., *Bears Guide to Earning Degrees By Distance*, 16, 2003

308 Kiyosaki, R. Lechter, S., *Rich Dad, Poor Dad*, 124, 2000

309 Moskowitz, M., *Standard of Living: The Measure of the Middle Class in Modern America*, 2004

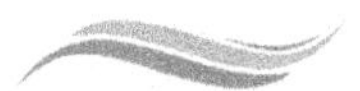

310 Bonner, W., Wiggin, A., *Empire of Debt: The Rise of An Epic Financial Crisis*, 2006

311 Meyer, A., *Evolution of United States Budgeting*, 39, 2002

312 Schweich, T., *Crashproof Your Life, A Comprehensive Three-Part Plan for Protecting Yourself from Financial Disaster*, 276, 2001

313 Kimbro, D., *What Makes The Great Great: Strategies for Extraordinary Achievement*, 215, 1997

314 Tracy, J., *Accounting for Dummies*, 84, 2001

315 Investors Group, *Starting Out: Smart Strategies for Your 20's and 30's*, 30, 1998

316 Magazine, *Black Enterprise, No Time Like The Present*, 113, Oct. 1999

317 Stanley, T., Danko, W., *The Millionaire Next Door: The Surprising Secrets of America's Wealthy*, 110, 1998

318 *Mobs, Messiahs, and Markets: Surviving The Public Spectacle in Finance and Politics*, 2007

319 Baumol, W., Blinder, A., *Economics: Principles and Policy*, 380, 2008

320 Givens, C., *Wealth Without Risk*, 508, 1995

321 *Consumer Reports, Used Car Buying Guide*, 10, 1998

322 General Motors, Volt Electric Car May Earn 250 mpg Rating, http://www.redorbit.com/news/business/1735849/volt_electric_car_may_earn_250_mpg_rating/index.html

323 Kelly, T., Tuccillio, J., *How a Second Home Can Be Your Best Investment*, 4, 2004

324 Strauss, S., Stone, M., *The Unofficial Guide To Real Estate Investing*, 2003

325 Lewis, N., *Gold: The Once and Future Money*, 2007

326 Bogle, J., Swenson, D., *Common Sense on Mutual Funds*, 149, 2009

327 Irwin, R., *Buy, Rent, and Sell: How To Profit By Investing In Real Estate*, 37, 2007

328 Campbell, C., *The Wealthy Spirit: Daily Affirmations For Financial Stress Reduction*, Introduction, 2002

329 Mosiah 4:27

330 Benson, E., *Beware of Pride, Ensign*, 4, May 1989

331 Oaks, D., *Why Do We Serve, Ensign*, 12, November 1984

332 Jackson, L., *Physical Appearance and Gender: Sociobiological and Sociocultural Perspectives*, 132, 1992

333 Moroni 7:48

334 Stamm, A., Harris, E., *Chemical Processing of Wood*, 374, 1953

335 Genesis 2:2,3

336 Mosiah 4:27

337 Franklin, B., *The Autobiography of Ben Franklin*, 2006

338 Nightingale, F., McDonald, L., *Florence Nightingale's Spiritual Journey: Biblical Annotations, Sermons, and Journal Notes*, 2002

339 Proverbs 3:6

SPIRIT SECTION:

340 Dickens, C., DeMille, A., *A Tale of Two Cities*, 569, 1922

341 Genesis 2:9

342 Kimball, S., *Tragedy or Destiny*, 1920

343 Movie, Oh God: Book II, 1980

344 2 Nephi 2:13

345 Tanner, N., *Thou Mayest Choose For Thyself*, Ensign, 7 Jul 1973

346 Hinckley, G., Wallace, M., *Standing For Something*, 128, 2001

347 Hinckley, G., Wallace, M., *Standing for Something*, 132, 2001

348 Hinckley, G., Wallace, M., *Standing For Something*, xxvii, 2001

349 FOX News, 92% of Americans Believe in God, November 20, 2009

350 FOX News, 67% of Americans Celebrate Christmas As The Birth of Christ, November 20, 2009

351 Galbraith, P., *Reversing Ageing*, 200, 1995

352 Hicks, E., Hicks, J., *The Law of Attraction, The Basics of the Teachings of Abraham*, 65, 2006

353 John 3:16

354 Psalms 94:11

355 Matthew 10:30

356 *A Parents Guide, Intimacy and The Purposes of Earthly Families*, 5, 2010

357 Psalms 119:30

358 Matthew 11:30

359 2 Samuel 23:3

360 Ephesians 4:32

361 Romans 2:11, Hebrews 13:8

362 Jeremiah 5:25

363 Tucker, L., What's On TV Tonight, *Ensign Magazine*, 18, 1988

364 Alma 41:10

365 Hebrews 5:9

366 Plato, The Republic, 608, 1976

367 Genesis Chapter 1

368 1 Corinthians 9:27

369 Joshua 24:15

370 Lockhart, B. *Mind/Body Fitness*, 1992

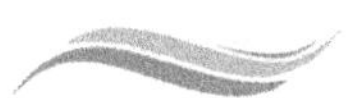

371 1 Corinthians 3:16

372 Panksepp, J., *Affective Neuroscience: The Foundations of Human and Animal Emotions*, 87, 2004

373 Galbraith, P., *Reversing Ageing*, 200, 1995

374 Matthew 17:20

375 Mark 9:23

376 Wilhelm, A., *Christ Among Us: A Modern Presentation of the Catholic Faith for Adults*, 37, 1996

377 Moses 5:18

378 Exodus 34:28

379 John 16:13

380 Psalms 82:6

381 Genesis 1:26

382 Moses 1:39

383 Revelation 21:7

384 Romans 12:1

385 Ehrman, B., *Lost Christianities: The Battles for Scripture and The Faith's We Never Knew*, 126, 2005

386 John 5:29

387 Hosea 13:14

388 Romans 8:17

389 1 Peter 3:18-20

390 Jeremiah 1:5

391 Luke 24:36-43

392 Matthew 27: 50-53

393 Romans 6:5

394 1 Corinthians 15:20-23

395 Alma 40:23

396 Philippians 3:21

397 2 Corinthians 3:18

398 Isaiah 53:2

399 *Family: A Proclamation to the World, Liahona Magazine*, 49, October, 2004

400 2 Corinthians 12:7-10

401 Luke 15:7

402 Moroni 7:47

403 1 Corinthians 13

404 1 Corinthians 12, 13

405 Alma 38:12

406 Galatians 5: 22
407 Maxwell, N., *Insights, Ensign Magazine*, 21, April 1974
408 1 John 3:2
409 Fireside attended by Tom, 1994
410 Find - 1996 there were 7 million fatherless families
411 Isaiah 53:3
412 Moroni 10:22
413 Matthew 24
414 Brezenski, S., *Little People Little Patriots: Saving America One Child at a Time*, 10, 1999
415 Alters, S., *Abortion: An Eternal Social and Moral Issue*, 98, 2006
416 McBride, D., *Abortion in the United States: A Reference Handbook*, 185, 2008
417 Alma 45: 16
418 Berman-Barrett, S., Bergman, P., *The Criminal Law Handbook: Survive The System*, 581, 2008
419 Proverbs 22:6
420 Matthew 5:48
421 Proverbs 13:15
422 Matthew 10:22
423 Sumner, T., *Roloff Family, Lessons in Love, Respect, and Understanding for Families of Any Size*, 41, 2008
424 Revelation 3:20
425 McKay, D., www.goodreads.com/author/quotes/601416.David O McKay
426 Hinckley, G., Wallace, M., *Standing For Something*, 256, 2001
427 Taffel, R., *Getting Through to Difficult Kids and Parents: Uncommon Sense for Child Professionals*, 125,
428 1 Thessalonians 5:18
429 Chariots of Fire movie, 1981
430 Matthew 25: 31-46
431 Revelation 7:15
432 Deuteronomy 16:17
433 Mosiah 4:19
434 Job 12:10
435 Luke 17:11-19
436 Psalms 104:24
437 Job 29:12
438 Moroni 7:48

WAVE 4 Healthy Living 2023

www.ingramcontent.com/pod-product-compliance
Lightning Source LLC
LaVergne TN
LVHW010601100826
845148LV00014B/2799

* 9 7 9 8 8 8 5 8 1 1 0 1 9 *